SPRINGHOUSE

Professional Care Guide

Infectious Disorders

Springhouse Corporation
Springhouse, Pennsylvania

Staff

Senior Publisher
Matthew Cahill

Clinical Manager
Cindy Tryniszewski, RN, MSN

Art Director
John Hubbard

Senior Editor
June Norris

Editors
Edith McMahon, Jane Cray, Elizabeth Weinstein

Clinical Editor
Beverly Tscheschlog, RN

Designers
Stephanie Peters (senior associate art director), Lynn Foulk (book designer)

Copy Editors
Cynthia C. Breuninger (manager), Lynette High, Doris Weinstock, Lewis Adams, Nancy Papsin

Typography
Diane Paluba (manager), Elizabeth Bergman, Joyce Rossi Biletz, Phyllis Marron, Robin Mayer, Valerie Rosenberger

Manufacturing
Deborah C. Meiris (director), Patricia Dorshaw, T.A. Landis

Production Coordinator
Patricia McCloskey

Editorial Assistants
Beverly Lane, Mary Madden, Dianne Tolbert

Indexer
Barbara Hodgson

The cover illustration depicts infection-causing microorganisms, including the AIDS, herpes simplex, and influenza viruses. The cover also shows viral invasion of a cell. Illustration by Kevin A. Somerville.

Contents

Contributors and Consultants

John G. Bartlett, MD
Professor of Medicine and
Chief, Infectious Diseases Division
The Johns Hopkins University
School of Medicine
Baltimore

Marlene M. Ciranowicz, RN, MSN, CDE
Independent Nurse Consultant
Dresher, Pa.

Judith E. Meissner, RN, MSN
Independent Nurse Consultant
Warminster, Pa.

Foreword

The history of infectious diseases in North America is replete with drama, unparalleled successes, and grim foreboding. Consider this brief chronology.

In the early 20th century, public health efforts effectively reduced infection rates for such incurable diseases as tuberculosis and cholera.

In the middle of the 20th century, the development of antibiotics brought about the greatest curative revolution in the history of medicine. Equally dramatic has been the story of vaccines, which have eradicated smallpox altogether and reduced the incidence of such diseases as polio, measles, and diphtheria by 98%.

Now, in the late 20th century, we are facing uncertainty. New pathogens, such as the human immunodeficiency virus (HIV), can't be treated successfully and there's little prospect of a vaccine. Bacteria are becoming increasingly resistant to antibiotics. In fact, many authorities believe that we're losing the war against microbes and anticipate a post-antibiotic era—a time when antibiotics are no longer effective. The forecast grows grimmer as newly recognized pathogens proliferate and infectious complications undercut medical progress, such as organ transplantation and immunosuppressive treatments.

Clearly, with this outlook, health care professionals need to be armed with up-to-date information and skills to serve them now and in the 21st century. To help them, they need accurate, practical, and trustworthy references, such as *Infectious Disorders*. Part of the Professional Care Guides series, this volume will help doctors, interns, nurses, and other health professionals provide expert care. It's up-to-date not only in its coverage of pathogens and their treatments but also in its ease of use in today's changing health care environment.

The book begins by examining the causes, diagnosis, and treatment of infection. Subsequent chapters address bacterial, viral, fungal, protozoal, and helminthic infections. A separate chapter covers additional infections, such as Rocky Mountain spotted fever and toxic shock syndrome. Lastly, the book's extensive appendices cover the full *ICD-9-CM* classification of infectious disorders and anti-infective drugs, including indications and adverse reactions.

For convenience, each disorder in the book's seven chapters is organized consistently. Each one covers causes, signs and symptoms, diagnostic studies, treatments, and special considerations. At the end of each chapter, you'll find a helpful self-test section. This section allows the reader to quickly evaluate understanding of the chapter's main concepts and clinical issues. Answers to these questions and the rationales appear at the back of the book.

Whether treatment occurs in a hospital, community, or long-term care setting, *Infectious Disorders* presents valuable diagnostic and therapeutic information. It will help the caregiver meet the patient's needs — quickly, effectively, and confidently.

John G. Bartlett, MD
Professor of Medicine and
Chief, Infectious Diseases Division
The Johns Hopkins University
School of Medicine
Baltimore

CHAPTER 1

Introduction

Despite improved methods of treating and preventing infection—potent antibiotics, complex immunizations, and modern sanitation—infection still accounts for many cases of serious illness, even in highly industrialized countries. In developing countries, infection remains one of the most critical health problems.

What is infection?

Infection is the invasion and multiplication of microorganisms in or on body tissue that produce signs and symptoms as well as an immune response. Such reproduction injures the host by causing cellular damage from microorganism-produced toxins or intracellular multiplication, or by competing with the host's metabolism. The host's own immune response may compound the tissue damage, which may be localized (as in infected pressure ulcers) or systemic. The severity of the infection varies with the pathogenicity and number of the invading microorganisms and the strength of the host's defenses.

Why are the microorganisms that cause infectious diseases so difficult to overcome? There are many complex reasons:
• Some bacteria develop a resistance to antibiotics.
• Some microorganisms—such as the influenza virus—include so many different strains that a single vaccine can't provide protection against them all.
• Most viruses resist antiviral drugs.
• Some microorganisms localize in areas that make treatment difficult. Examples of such areas are the central nervous system and bone.

Moreover, certain factors that contribute to improved health—such as the affluence that allows good nutrition and living conditions, and advances in medical science—can increase the risk of infection. For example, travel can expose persons to diseases for which they have little natural immunity. The expanded use of immunosuppressants, surgery, and other invasive procedures also increases the risk of in-

Epidemiology defined

The dynamic study of various factors as they relate to the occurrence, frequency, and distribution of disease in a given population is called epidemiology. It includes the origin of the disease, how it's transmitted, and host and environmental factors that influence the development of the disease.

Several terms describe the occurrence or frequency of a disease. In an *epidemic,* a disease occurs at a level that is higher than normal. An *outbreak,* however, is a sudden appearance of the disease, often in a small portion of the population. An *endemic* disease is persistently present in a given locale; a *hyperendemic* disease is persistent and has a high incidence.

Reservoir refers to the natural habitat of the organism responsible for the disease; *source,* to the site (or milieu) from which the host directly acquires the disease. Infectious organisms can multiply within the source. A source may be a *vector,* an animal or insect (such as a mosquito) that acts as an intermediary between two or more hosts in the transmission of infection. Or it may be a person who has the disease, was recently exposed to it, or is a carrier. Transmission may also occur through a *vehicle,* such as contaminated food or water, within which infectious organisms can multiply.

---

fection. (See *Epidemiology defined* and *Reportable infectious diseases.*)

Types of infections

A laboratory-verified infection that causes no signs and symptoms is called a subclinical, silent, or asymptomatic infection. A multiplication of microbes that produces no signs, symptoms, or immune responses is called a colonization. A person with a subclinical infection or colonization may be a carrier and transmit infection to others. A latent infection occurs after a microorganism has been dormant in the host, sometimes for years. An exogenous infection results from environmental pathogens; an endogenous infection, from the host's normal flora. (For instance, *Escherichia coli* displaced from the colon causes a urinary tract infection.)

The varied forms of microorganisms responsible for infectious diseases include bacteria, viruses, rickettsiae, chlamydiae, fungi (yeasts and molds), and protozoa; larger organisms, such as helminths (worms), may also cause disease.

Bacteria

Single-cell microorganisms with well-defined cell walls, bacteria can grow independently on artificial media without

Reportable infectious diseases

Because disease reporting laws vary from state to state, this list isn't conclusive and may change periodically. Local agencies report certain diseases to state health departments, which in turn determine which diseases are reported to the Centers for Disease Control and Prevention.

- [ ] Acquired immunodeficiency syndrome
- [ ] Amebiasis
- [ ] Animal bites
- [ ] Anthrax (cutaneous or pulmonary)
- [ ] Arbovirus
- [ ] Aseptic meningitis
- [ ] Botulism
- [ ] Brucellosis
- [ ] Campylobacteriosis
- [ ] Chancroid
- [ ] Chlamydial infections
- [ ] Cholera
- [ ] Diarrhea of the newborn (epidemic)
- [ ] Diphtheria (cutaneous or pharyngeal)
- [ ] Encephalitis (postinfectious or primary)
- [ ] Food poisoning
- [ ] Gastroenteritis (hospital outbreak)
- [ ] Giardiasis
- [ ] Gonococcal infections
- [ ] Gonorrhea
- [ ] Group A beta-hemolytic streptococcal infections (including scarlet fever)
- [ ] Guillain-Barré syndrome
- [ ] Hepatitis A
- [ ] Hepatitis B
- [ ] Hepatitis C (formerly called non-A, non-B)
- [ ] Hepatitis (unspecified)
- [ ] Histoplasmosis
- [ ] Influenza
- [ ] Kawasaki disease
- [ ] Lead poisoning
- [ ] *Legionella* infections (Legionnaires' disease)
- [ ] Leprosy
- [ ] Leptospirosis
- [ ] Listeriosis
- [ ] Lyme disease
- [ ] Lymphogranuloma venereum
- [ ] Malaria
- [ ] Measles
- [ ] Meningitis
- [ ] Meningococcal disease
- [ ] Mumps
- [ ] Neonatal hypothyroidism
- [ ] Pertussis
- [ ] Phenylketonuria
- [ ] Plague
- [ ] Poliomyelitis
- [ ] Psittacosis
- [ ] Rabies
- [ ] Reye's syndrome
- [ ] Rheumatic fever
- [ ] Rickettsial diseases (including Rocky Mountain spotted fever)
- [ ] Rubella and congenital rubella syndrome
- [ ] Salmonellosis (excluding typhoid fever)
- [ ] Shigellosis
- [ ] Staphylococcal infections (neonatal)
- [ ] Syphilis (congenital under age 1)
- [ ] Syphilis (primary or secondary)
- [ ] Tetanus
- [ ] Toxic shock syndrome
- [ ] Toxoplasmosis
- [ ] Trichinosis
- [ ] Tuberculosis
- [ ] Tularemia
- [ ] Typhoid and paratyphoid fever
- [ ] Typhus
- [ ] Varicella
- [ ] Yellow fever

the need for other cells. In developing countries, where poor sanitation potentiates infection, bacterial infections are common causes of death and disability. In industrialized countries, they're the most common fatal infections.

Bacteria can be classified according to shape. Spherical bacteria are called *cocci;* rod-shaped bacteria, *bacilli;* and spiral-shaped bacteria, *spirilla.* They can also be classified according to their response to staining (gram-positive, gram-negative, or acid-fast bacteria), their motility (motile or nonmotile bacteria), tendency to capsulation (encapsulated or nonencapsulated bacteria), and their capacity to form spores (sporulating or nonsporulating bacteria).

Spirochetes are bacteria with flexible, slender, undulating spiral rods that have cell walls. Most are anaerobic. The three forms that are pathogenic in humans include *Treponema, Leptospira,* and *Borrelia.*

Viruses

These subcellular microorganisms consist of a ribonucleic acid or deoxyribonucleic acid nucleus covered with proteins. They're the smallest known microorganisms. Independent of host cells, viruses can't replicate. Rather, they invade a host cell and stimulate it to participate in the formation of additional virus particles. The estimated 400 viruses that infect humans are classified according to their size, shape (spherical, rod-shaped, or cubic), or means of transmission (respiratory, fecal, oral, or sexual).

Rickettsiae

Relatively uncommon in North America, these small, gram-negative, bacteria-like microorganisms frequently induce life-threatening infections. Like viruses, they require a host cell for replication. Three genera of rickettsiae include *Rickettsia, Coxiella,* and *Rochalimaea.*

Chlamydiae

Smaller than rickettsiae and bacteria but larger than viruses, chlamydiae depend on host cells for replication. Unlike viruses, they're susceptible to antibiotics.

Fungi

These single-cell microorganisms have nuclei enveloped by membranes. Fungi have rigid cell walls, like plant cells, but lack chlorophyll, the green matter necessary for photosynthesis; they also exhibit relatively little cellular specialization. Fungi occur as yeasts (single-cell, oval-shaped organisms) or molds (organisms with hyphae, or branching filaments). Depending on the environment, some fungi may occur in both forms. Fungal diseases in humans are called mycosis.

Protozoa

The simplest single-cell organisms of the animal kingdom, protozoa exhibit a high level of cellular specialization. Like other animal cells, they have cell membranes rather than cell walls, and their nuclei are surrounded by nuclear membranes.

Larger parasites

Infectious diseases may also result from larger parasites, including roundworms and flatworms.

Modes of transmission

Most infectious diseases are transmitted in one of four ways.
• In contact transmission, the susceptible host comes into direct contact (as in venereal disease) or indirect contact (through contaminated inanimate objects) with the source.
• Airborne transmission results from inhalation of contaminated aerosolized droplets (as in pulmonary tuberculosis).
• In enteric (oral-fecal) transmission, the infecting organisms are found in feces and are ingested by susceptible victims, often through fecally contaminated food or water (as in salmonella infections).
• Vector-borne transmission occurs when an intermediate carrier (vector), such as a flea or a mosquito, transfers an organism.

Much can be done to prevent transmission of infectious diseases:
• comprehensive immunization (including the required immunization of people traveling to or from endemic areas)
• drug prophylaxis
• improved nutrition, living conditions, and sanitation
• correction of environmental factors.

Immunization can now control many diseases, including diphtheria, tetanus, pertussis, measles, rubella, some forms of meningitis, poliovirus, hepatitis B, pneumococcal pneumonia, influenza, rabies, and tetanus. Smallpox (variola)—which killed and disfigured millions in the early part of this century—is believed to have been successfully eradicated by a comprehensive World Health Organization pro-

Immunization schedule

Childhood immunizations are usually given on the fixed schedule described below. Before immunization, obtain the child's medication, illness, and allergy history. Instruct parents to report a severe reaction to the vaccine.

AGE	IMMUNIZATION
Birth	Hepatitis B (HBV) vaccine
1 to 2 months	HBV vaccine
2 months	First dose: diphtheria, pertussis, tetanus (DPT) vaccine; oral polio vaccine (OPV); haemophilus b conjugate vaccine (HbCV)
4 months	Second dose: DPT vaccine, OPV, and HbCV
6 months	Third dose: DPT vaccine and OPV (optional), and HbCV
6 to 18 months	HBV vaccine
12 months	HbCV
15 months	Measles, mumps, rubella (MMR) vaccine; HbCV
18 months	DPT vaccine; OPV
4 to 6 years	DPT vaccine; OPV
11 to 12 years	MMR vaccine
14 to 16 years	Tetanus and diphtheria toxoids

gram of surveillance and immunization. (See *Immunization schedule.*)

Vaccines – which contain live but attenuated (weakened) or killed microorganisms – and toxoids – which contain modified bacterial exotoxins – induce active immunity against bacterial and viral diseases by stimulating antibody formation. Immune serums contain previously formed antibodies from hyperimmunized donors or pooled plasma and provide temporary passive immunity. Antitoxins provide passive immunity to various toxins. Generally, passive immunization is used only when active immunization is perilous or impossible or when complete protection requires both active and passive immunization.

Although prophylactic antibiotic therapy may prevent certain diseases, the risk of superinfection and the emergence of drug-resistant strains may outweigh the benefits. So prophylactic antibiotics are usually reserved for patients at high risk for exposure to dangerous infections. Antibiotic-resistant bacteria are on the rise mainly because antibiotics have been misused and overused. Some bacteria, such as enterococci, have developed mutant strains that do not respond to antibiotic therapy.

Nosocomial infections

A nosocomial infection develops after a patient is admitted to a hospital or another institution. This type of infection is usually transmitted by direct contact. Less frequently, it results from inhalation or from contact with contaminated equipment or solutions.

Despite hospital programs of infection control that include surveillance, prevention, and education, about 5% of patients who enter hospitals contract a nosocomial infection. Since the 1960s, staphylococcal infections have been declining; however, gram-negative bacilli and fungal infections have been steadily increasing.

Nosocomial infections continue to be a difficult problem because most hospital patients are older and more debilitated than in the past. Moreover, the increased use of invasive and surgical procedures, immunosuppressants, and antibiotics predisposes patients to infection and superinfection. At the same time, the growing number of personnel who can come in contact with each patient makes the risk of exposure greater.

Here's how you can prevent nosocomial infections:
• Follow strict infection control procedures.
• Document hospital infections as they occur.
• Identify outbreaks early and take steps to prevent their spread.
• Eliminate unnecessary procedures that contribute to infection.
• Strictly follow necessary isolation guidelines. (See *Transmission prevention guidelines,* pages 8 to 10.)
• Observe *all* patients for signs of infection, especially those at high risk.
• Follow good hand-washing technique, and encourage other staff members to do the same.
• Keep staff and visitors with obvious infection, as well as known carriers, away from susceptible patients.

Transmission prevention guidelines

To prevent the transmission of infectious diseases in hospitals and other clinical settings, the Centers for Disease Control and Prevention has established a category-specific isolation system, which classifies six of its seven categories of isolation precautions according to major modes of transmission. The seventh category, universal precautions, has been expanded to cover *all* patients—not just those with known or suspected blood-borne diseases. Because of the special concern about the risk of transmitting human immunodeficiency virus, this category is covered separately.

TYPE OF ISOLATION AND DISEASES REQUIRING ISOLATION	PRIVATE ROOM	MASK	GOWN	GLOVES	SPECIAL HANDLING
Strict isolation Prevents transmission of contagious or virulent infections by air or contact. Special ventilation is required. *Diseases:* pharyngeal diphtheria, viral hemorrhagic fevers, pneumonic plague, smallpox, varicella-zoster virus (localized in immunocompromised patient or disseminated)	X with door closed	X	X	X	X
Contact isolation Prevents transmission of epidemiologically important infections that don't require strict isolation. Health care workers should wear masks, gowns, and gloves for direct or close contact, depending on the infection. *Diseases in any age-group:* group A streptococcal endometritis; impetigo; pediculosis; *Staphylococcus aureus* or *Streptococcus pneumoniae* infection; rabies; rubella; scabies; staphylococcal scalded skin syndrome; major skin, wound, or burn infection (draining and not adequately covered by dressing); vaccinia; primary disseminated herpes simplex; cutaneous diphtheria; infection or colonization with bacteria that resist antibiotic therapy *Diseases in infants and young children:* acute respiratory infections, influenza, infectious pharyngitis, viral pneumonia, group A streptococcal infection *Diseases in neonates:* gonococcal conjunctivitis, staphylococcal furunculosis, neonatal disseminated herpes simplex	X	O	S	S	X

Transmission prevention guidelines *(continued)*

TYPE OF ISOLATION AND DISEASES REQUIRING ISOLATION	PRIVATE ROOM	MASK	GOWN	GLOVES	SPECIAL HANDLING
Respiratory isolation Prevents transmission of infections spread primarily through the air by droplets ***Diseases:*** *Haemophilus influenzae* epiglottitis, erythema infectiosum, measles, *H. influenzae* or meningococcal pneumonia, meningococcemia, mumps, pertussis	X with door closed	X	–	–	X
Acid-fast bacillus isolation Prevents patient with active pulmonary or laryngeal tuberculosis from transmitting acid-fast bacillus to other patients. Patient requires special ventilation. ***Disease:*** tuberculosis	X with door closed	X*	S	–	X
Enteric precautions Prevent transmission of infection through direct or indirect contact with feces ***Diseases:*** amebic dysentery; cholera; coxsackievirus disease; acute diarrhea with suspected infection; echovirus disease; encephalitis (unless known not to be caused by enteroviruses); *Clostridium difficile* or enterocolitis caused by *Staphylococcus;* enteroviral infection; gastroenteritis caused by *Campylobacter* species, *Cryptosporidium* species, *Dientamoeba fragilis, Escherichia coli, Giardia lamblia, Salmonella* species, *Shigella* species, *Vibrio parahaemolyticus,* viruses, or *Yersinia enterocolitica;* hand-foot-and-mouth disease; hepatitis A; herpangina; necrotizing enterocolitis; pleurodynia; poliomyelitis; typhoid fever; viral pericarditis, viral myocarditis, and viral meningitis (unless known not to be caused by enteroviruses)	D	–	S	S	X

(continued)

Transmission prevention guidelines *(continued)*

TYPE OF ISOLATION AND DISEASES REQUIRING ISOLATION	PRIVATE ROOM	MASK	GOWN	GLOVES	SPECIAL HANDLING
Drainage and secretion precautions Prevent transmission of infection from direct or indirect contact with purulent material or drainage **Diseases:** conjunctivitis; minor or limited abscess; minor or limited burn, skin, wound, or pressure ulcer infection; herpes zoster (shingles)	–	–	S	S	X

Key
X = Always necessary
S = Necessary if soiling of hands or clothing is likely
O = Necessary for close contact or if patient is coughing and doesn't reliably cover mouth
D = Desirable but optional; necessary only if patient has poor hygiene

*Mask must be particulate respirator

• Take special precautions with vulnerable patients—those with indwelling urinary catheters, mechanical ventilators, or I.V. lines, and those recuperating from surgery. (See *Universal precautions.*)

Accurate evaluation vital

Complete, accurate patient evaluation helps identify infectious diseases and prevents avoidable complications. Such evaluation consists of a patient history, a physical examination, and laboratory data. The history should include the patient's sex, age, address, occupation, and place of work; known exposure to illness; and date of disease onset. It should also detail information about recent hospitalization, blood transfusions, blood donation denial by the American Red Cross or other agencies, vaccination, travel or camping trips, and exposure to animals. If applicable, ask about possible exposure to sexually transmitted diseases and about drug abuse. Also, try to determine the patient's resistance to infectious disease. Ask about dietary patterns, unusual fatigue, and any conditions, such as neoplastic disease or alcoholism, that may predispose him to infection. Note whether the patient is listless or uneasy, lacks concentration, or has any obvious abnormality of mood or affect.

If you suspect infection, a physical examination assessing the skin, mucous membranes, liver, spleen, and lymph

Universal precautions

The Centers for Disease Control and Prevention recommends that universal blood and body-fluid precautions be used for *all* patients. This is especially important in emergency care settings, where the risk of blood exposure is increased and the patient's infection status is usually unknown. Implementation of universal precautions doesn't eliminate the need for other category- or disease-specific isolation precautions, such as enteric precautions for infectious diarrhea or acid-fast bacillus isolation precautions for pulmonary tuberculosis.

Sources of potential exposure

Universal precautions apply to blood, semen, vaginal secretions, cerebrospinal fluid, synovial fluid, pleural fluid, peritoneal fluid, pericardial fluid, and amniotic fluid. These fluids are most likely to transmit human immunodeficiency virus (HIV). Universal precautions also apply to other body fluids—including feces, nasal secretions, saliva, sputum, sweat, tears, vomitus, and breast milk.

Barrier precautions

• Wear gloves when touching blood and body fluids, mucous membranes, or broken skin of all patients; when handling items or touching surfaces soiled with blood or body fluids; and when performing venipuncture and other vascular access procedures.
• Change gloves and wash hands after contact with each patient.
• Wear a mask and protective eyewear or a face shield to protect mucous membranes of the mouth, nose, and eyes during procedures that may generate blood drops or other body fluids.

• Wear a gown or an apron during procedures that are likely to generate splashing of blood or other body fluids.
• After removing gloves, thoroughly wash hands and other skin surfaces that may be contaminated with blood, body fluids containing visible blood, or other body fluids to which universal precautions apply.

Precautions for invasive procedures

• During all invasive procedures, wear gloves, a surgical mask and goggles, or a face shield.
• During procedures that commonly generate droplets or splashes of blood or other body fluids, or that generate bone chips, wear protective eyewear and a mask, or a face shield.
• During invasive procedures that are likely to cause splashing or splattering of blood or other body fluids, wear a gown or an impervious apron.
• If you perform or assist in vaginal or cesarean deliveries, wear gloves and a gown when handling the placenta or the infant and during umbilical cord care.

Work practice precautions

Prevent injuries caused by needles, scalpels, and other sharp instruments or devices when cleaning used instruments, when disposing of used needles, and when handling sharp instruments after procedures.
• To prevent needle-stick injuries, do not recap used needles, bend or break needles, remove them from disposable syringes, or manipulate them.
• Place disposable syringes and needles, scalpel blades, and other sharp items in puncture-resistant containers for disposal, making sure these contain-

(continued)

Universal precautions   *(continued)*

ers are located near the area of use.
• Place large-bore reusable needles in a puncture-resistant container for transport to the reprocessing area.
• If a glove tears or a needle-stick or other injury occurs, remove the glove and put on a new one as quickly as patient safety permits; remove the needle or instrument involved in the incident from the sterile field. Promptly report needle-stick injuries and mucous-membrane exposure to the appropriate infection-control officer.

Additional precautions
• Make sure mouthpieces, one-way valve masks, resuscitation bags, or other ventilation devices are available in areas where the need for resuscitation is likely. *Note:* Saliva has not been implicated in HIV transmission.
• If you have exudative lesions or weeping dermatitis, refrain from direct patient care and handling patient care equipment until the condition resolves.

nodes is essential. Check for and note the location and type of drainage from skin lesions. Record skin color, temperature, and turgor. Ask the patient if he has pruritus. Take his temperature, using the same route consistently, and note whether he has a fever. (Fever is the best indicator of many infections.) Note and record the pattern of temperature change and the effect of antipyretics. Be aware that certain analgesics may contain antipyretics. In cases of high fever, especially in children, watch for seizures.

Check the patient's pulse rate. Infection often increases pulse rate; however, some infections, notably typhoid fever and psittacosis, may decrease it. In cases of severe infection or when complications are possible, watch for hypotension, hematuria, oliguria, hepatomegaly, jaundice, bleeding from gums or into joints, and altered level of consciousness.

Obtain laboratory studies and appropriate cultures. (See *How to collect culture specimens.*)

How to collect culture specimens

Proper identification of the causative organism requires proper culture collection. Label the culture specimen with the date, time, patient's name, suspected diagnosis, and source of culture.

CULTURE SITE	SPECIMEN SOURCE	SPECIAL CONSIDERATIONS
Infected wound	• Aspiration of exudate with syringe (preferred technique)	• Use only sterile syringe. Pungent odor suggests the presence of anaerobes. Use oxygen-free collection tubes if available.
	• Applicator swab	• Firmly but gently insert swab deep into wound and saturate it with exudate from infected site. If surface is dry, moisten swab with sterile saline solution before taking culture.
Skin lesions	• Excision or puncture	• Thoroughly clean skin before excision or puncture, and follow procedure for infected wound.
Eye	• Cotton swab	• Carefully retract lower lid and gently swab conjunctiva.
	• Corneal scrapings	• Use a swab loop to scrape specimen from site of corneal infection. Reassure patient that procedure is short and discomfort minimal.
Upper respiratory tract	• Nasopharyngeal swab (generally used to detect carriers of *Staphylococcus aureus* and viral infections)	• Gently pass swab through nose into nasopharynx. Immediately send specimen to laboratory for culture.
	• Throat swab	• Under adequate light, swab inflamed or exudative area .
Lower respiratory tract	• Expectorated sputum	• Instruct patient to cough deeply and to expectorate into cup. Culture requires expectorated sputum, not just saliva from mouth.
	• Induced sputum (used when patient can't expectorate sputum)	• Use aerosol mist spray of saline solution or water to induce sputum production. Apply cupping and postural drainage if needed.
	• Nasotracheal suction	• Measure approximate distance from patient's nose to his ear. Note the distance; then, insert a sterile suction catheter this length, with a collection vial attached, into his nose. Maintain suction during catheter withdrawal.
	• Pleural tap	• Advise patient that he may feel discomfort even though skin is anesthetized before this procedure. After tap, check site often for local swelling, and be alert for dyspnea and other adverse reactions.

(continued)

How to collect culture specimens *(continued)*

CULTURE SITE	SPECIMEN SOURCE	SPECIAL CONSIDERATIONS
Lower intestinal tract	• Rectal swab	• Lesion on colon or on rectal wall may require colonoscopy or sigmoidoscopy to obtain specimen. If so, explain the procedure. Help patient to assume a left lateral decubitus or a knee-chest position.
	• Stool specimen	• Specimen should contain any pus or blood present in feces and a sampling of the first, middle, and last portion of stools. Urine with stools can invalidate results. Immediately send specimen to laboratory in a clean, tightly covered container, especially stools being examined for ova and parasites.
Genital tract	• Swab specimen	• In males, specimen should contain urethral discharge or prostatic fluid; in females, urethral or cervical specimens. Always collect specimens on two swabs simultaneously.
Urinary tract	• Midstream, clean-catch urine specimen (avoids specimen contamination with microorganisms commonly found in the lower urethra and perineum)	• In an uninfected person, midstream, clean-catch specimen should contain less than 10,000 bacteria/ml. • Teach patient how to collect specimen or supervise collection. In males, retract foreskin and clean glans penis; in females, clean and separate labia so urinary meatus is clearly visible; then clean meatus. Tell patient to void 25 to 30 ml and, without stopping urine stream, to collect specimen. • In infants, apply collection bag carefully and check it frequently to avoid mechanical urethral obstruction. • Immediately send urine to laboratory or refrigerate it to retard growth.
	• Indwelling urinary catheter specimen	• Clean specimen port of catheter with alcohol, and aspirate urine with a sterile needle or from a latex catheter, at a point distal to the "Y" branch.
Body fluids	• Needle aspiration	• Immediately send peritoneal and synovial fluid and cerebrospinal fluid (CSF) to laboratory. *Don't* retard growth of CSF organisms by refrigerating specimen. After pericardial and pleural fluid aspiration, observe patient carefully and check vital signs often. Watch for signs of pneumothorax or cardiac tamponade.
Blood	• Venous or arterial aspiration	• Prepare skin according to your hospital's policy. • Using a sterile syringe, collect 12 to 15 ml blood, changing needles before injecting blood into aerobic and anaerobic collection bottles. Continue procedure according to your hospital's policy. • If patient is receiving antibiotics, note this on laboratory slip, because laboratory may add enzymes or resins to culture to inactivate drug.

Self-test questions

You can quickly review your comprehension of this introductory chapter by answering the following questions. The correct answers to these questions and their rationales appear on pages 186 and 187.

1. Which of the following statements correctly characterizes infection?
   a. Infection remains one of the most critical health care problems, even in highly industrialized countries.
   b. Infection results from the invasion of body tissue by microorganisms that subsequently multiply with or without activating an immune response.
   c. The severity of infection varies with the pathogenicity and number of invading microorganisms and the strength of host defenses.
   d. Bacterial infections are hard to overcome because most species develop a resistance to antibiotics.

2. A symptomatic urinary tract infection caused by *Escherichia coli* is an example of:
   a. a subclinical infection.
   b. a latent infection.
   c. an exogenous infection.
   d. an endogenous infection.

3. Which of the following classes is made up of the simplest single-cell organisms of the animal kingdom?
   a. Bacteria
   b. Chlamydiae
   c. Fungi
   d. Protozoa

4. The transmission of an infectious microorganism by an intermediate carrier is called:
   a. indirect contact transmission.
   b. airborne transmission.
   c. oral-fecal transmission.
   d. vector-borne transmission.

5. Nosocomial infection is usually transmitted by:
   a. direct contact.
   b. indirect contact with contaminated equipment.
   c. air.
   d. the enteric route.

6. The most reliable indicator of many infections is:
   a. skin color and turgor.
   b. body temperature.
   c. pulse rate.
   d. blood pressure.

CHAPTER 2

Bacterial Infections

The microorganisms that cause bacterial infections include gram-positive and gram-negative cocci, gram-positive and gram-negative bacilli, spirochetes, and mycobacteria.

GRAM-POSITIVE COCCI

Although most gram-positive cocci cause organ-specific disorders, *Staphylococcus aureus* and group A beta-hemolytic streptococci cause systemic disorders.

Staphylococcal infections include bacteremia, pneumonia, osteomyelitis, enterocolitis, food poisoning, and skin infections (see *Staphylococcal infections*, pages 18 and 19).

Streptococcal infections include streptococcal pharyngitis, impetigo, bacterial endocarditis, scarlet fever, erysipelas, streptococcal gangrene, neonatal streptococcal infections, adult group B streptococcal infection, and otitis media (see *Streptococcal infections*, pages 20 to 22).

Staphylococcal infections

Staphylococci are coagulase-negative *(S. epidermidis)* or coagulase-positive *(S. aureus)* gram-positive bacteria. Coagulase-negative staphylococci, which grow abundantly as normal flora on skin and in the upper respiratory tract, are usually nonpathogenic but can cause serious infections. Pathogenic strains of staphylococci are found in many adult "carriers" — usually on the nasal mucosa, axilla, or groin. Sometimes, carriers shed staphylococci, infecting themselves or other susceptible people. Coagulase-positive staphylococci tend to form pus; they cause many types of infections.

PREDISPOSING FACTORS	SIGNS AND SYMPTOMS	DIAGNOSIS
Enterocolitis • Broad-spectrum antibiotics (tetracycline, chloramphenicol, or neomycin) as prophylaxis for bowel surgery or treatment of hepatic coma • Usually occurs in elderly people, but also in newborns (associated with staphylococcal skin lesions)	• Sudden onset of profuse, watery diarrhea usually 2 days to several weeks after start of antibiotic therapy, I.V. or P.O. • Nausea, vomiting, abdominal pain and distention • Hypovolemia and dehydration (decreased skin turgor, hypotension, fever)	• Stool Gram stain: many gram-positive cocci and polymorphonuclear leukocytes, with few gram-negative rods • Stool culture: *S. aureus* • Sigmoidoscopy: mucosal ulcerations • Blood studies: leukocytosis, moderately increased blood urea nitrogen level, and decreased serum albumin level
Food poisoning • Enterotoxin produced by toxogenic strains of *S. aureus* in contaminated food (second most common cause of food poisoning in United States)	• Anorexia, nausea, vomiting, diarrhea, and abdominal cramps 1 to 6 hours after ingestion of contaminated food • Symptoms usually subside within 18 hours, with complete recovery in 1 to 3 days.	• Clinical findings sufficient. • Stool cultures usually negative for *S. aureus*.
Skin infections • Decreased resistance • Burns or pressure ulcers • Decreased blood flow • Possible skin contamination from nasal discharge • Foreign bodies • Underlying skin diseases, such as eczema and acne • Common in persons with poor hygiene living in crowded quarters	• Cellulitis — diffuse, acute inflammation of soft tissue (no drainage) • Pus-producing lesions in and around hair follicles (folliculitis) • Boil-like lesions (furuncles and carbuncles) extend from hair follicles to subcutaneous tissues. These painful, red, indurated lesions are 1 to 2 cm and have a purulent yellow discharge. • Small macule or skin bleb that may develop into vesicle containing pus (bullous impetigo); common in school-age children • Mild or spiking fever • Malaise	• Clinical findings and analysis of pus cultures if sites are draining • Cultures of nondraining cellulitis taken from the margin of the reddened area by infiltration with 1 ml sterile saline solution and immediate fluid aspiration

TREATMENT	SPECIAL CONSIDERATIONS
• Broad-spectrum antibiotics should be discontinued. • Antistaphylococcal agents, such as vancomycin P.O., may be given.	• Monitor vital signs frequently to prevent shock. Force fluids to correct dehydration. • Know serum electrolyte levels. Measure and record bowel movements when possible. Check serum chloride level for alkalosis (hypochloremia). • Collect serial stool specimens for Gram stain, and culture for diagnosis and for evaluating effectiveness of treatment.
• No treatment necessary unless dehydration becomes a problem (usually in infants and elderly people); then, I.V. therapy may be necessary to replace fluids	• Obtain a complete history of symptoms, recent meals, and other known cases of food poisoning. • Monitor vital signs, fluid balance, and serum electrolyte levels. • Check for dehydration, if vomiting is severe or prolonged, and for decreased blood pressure. • Observe and report the number and color of stools.
• Topical ointments; bacitracin-neomycin-polymyxin or gentamicin • P.O. cloxacillin, dicloxacillin, or erythromycin; I.V. oxacillin or nafcillin for severe infection; I.V. vancomycin for oxacillin-resistant organisms • Application of heat to reduce pain • Surgical drainage • Identification and treatment of sources of reinfection (nostrils, perineum) • Cleaning and covering the area with moist, sterile dressings	• Identify the site and extent of infection. • Keep lesions clean with saline solution and peroxide irrigations as ordered. Cover infections near wounds or genitourinary tract with gauze pads. Keep pressure off the site to facilitate healing. • Be alert for the extension of skin infections. • Severe infection or abscess may require surgical drainage. Explain the procedure to the patient. Determine if cultures will be taken, and be ready to collect a specimen. • Impetigo is contagious. Isolate the patient and alert his family. Use secretion precautions for all draining lesions.

Streptococcal infections

Streptococci are small gram-positive bacteria linked together in pairs of chains. Although researchers have identified 21 species of streptococci, three classes — groups A, B, and D — cause most of the infections. When streptococci cause infection, drainage tends to be thin and serous.

CAUSES AND INCIDENCE	SIGNS AND SYMPTOMS
S. pyogenes (group A streptococci)	
Scarlet fever (scarlatina) • Usually follows streptococcal pharyngitis; may follow wound infections or puerperal sepsis • Caused by streptococcal strain that releases an erythrogenic toxin • Most common in children ages 2 to 10 • Spread by inhalation or direct contact	• Streptococcal sore throat, fever, strawberry tongue, fine erythematous rash that blanches on pressure and resembles sunburn with goosebumps • Rash usually appears first on upper chest, then spreads to neck, abdomen, legs, and arms, sparing soles and palms; flushed cheeks, pallor around mouth • Skin sheds during convalescence.
Erysipelas • Occurs primarily in infants and adults over age 30 • Usually follows strep throat • Exact mode of spread to skin unknown	• Sudden onset, with reddened, swollen, raised lesions (skin looks like an orange peel), usually on face and scalp, bordered by areas that often contain easily ruptured blebs filled with yellow-tinged fluid. Lesions sting and itch. Lesions on the trunk, arms, or legs usually affect incision or wound sites. • Other symptoms: vomiting, fever, headache, cervical lymphadenopathy, sore throat
Streptococcal gangrene (necrotizing fasciitis) • More common in elderly people with arteriosclerotic vascular disease or diabetes • Predisposing factors: surgery, wounds, skin ulcers • Spread by direct contact	• Mimics gas gangrene; within 72 hours of onset, patient shows red-streaked, painful skin lesion with dusky red surrounding tissue. Bullae with yellow or reddish black fluid develop and rupture. • Other symptoms: fever, tachycardia, lethargy, prostration, disorientation, hypotension, jaundice, hypovolemia, severe pain followed by anesthesia (due to nerve destruction)
S. agalactiae (group B streptococci)	
Neonatal streptococcal infections • Incidence of early-onset infection (age 5 days or less): 2/1,000 live births • Incidence of late-onset infection (age 7 days to 3 months): 1/1,000 live births • Spread by vaginal delivery or hands of nursery staff • Predisposing factors: maternal genital tract colonization, membrane rupture over 24 hours before delivery, crowded nursery	• Early onset: bacteremia, pneumonia, and meningitis; mortality from 14% for infants over 1,500 g at birth to 61% for infants under 1,500 g at birth • Late onset: bacteremia with meningitis, fever, and bone and joint involvement; mortality 15% to 20% • Other symptoms, such as skin lesions, depend on the site affected.

DIAGNOSIS	COMPLICATIONS	TREATMENT AND SPECIAL CONSIDERATIONS
• Characteristic rash and strawberry tongue • Culture and Gram stain show *S. pyogenes* from nasopharynx. • Granulocytosis	• Although rare, complications may include high fever, arthritis, and jaundice.	• Penicillin or erythromycin • Isolation for first 24 hours • Carefully dispose of purulent discharge. • Stress the need for prompt and complete antibiotic treatment.
• Typical reddened lesions • Culture taken from edge of lesions shows group A beta-hemolytic streptococci. • Throat culture is almost always positive for group A beta-hemolytic streptococci.	• Untreated lesions on trunk, arms, or legs may involve large body areas and lead to death.	• Penicillin I.V. or P.O. • Cold packs, analgesics (aspirin and codeine for local discomfort) • Prevention: prompt treatment of streptococcal infections and drainage and secretion precautions
• Culture and Gram stain usually show *S. pyogenes* from early bullous lesions and frequently from blood.	• Extensive necrotic sloughing • Bacteremia, metastatic abscesses, and death • Thrombophlebitis, when lower extremities are involved	• Immediate, wide, deep surgery of all necrotic tissues • High-dose penicillin I.V. • Good preoperative skin preparation; aseptic surgical and suturing technique
• Isolation of group B streptococci from blood, cerebrospinal fluid (CSF), or skin • Chest X-ray shows massive infiltrate similar to that of respiratory distress syndrome or pneumonia.	• Overwhelming pneumonia, sepsis, and death	• Penicillin or ampicillin I.V. • Patient isolation is unnecessary unless open draining lesion is present, but careful hand washing is essential. If draining lesion is present, take drainage and secretion precautions. • Vaccine is in developmental stages.

(continued)

Streptococcal infections *(continued)*

CAUSES AND INCIDENCE	SIGNS AND SYMPTOMS
S. agalactiae (group B streptococci) *(continued)*	
Adult group B streptococcal infection • Most adult infections occur in postpartum women, usually in the form of endometritis or wound infection following cesarean section. • Incidence of group B streptococcal endometritis: 1.3 per 1,000 live births	• Fever, malaise, uterine tenderness
S. pneumoniae (group D streptococci)	
Pneumococcal pneumonia • Accounts for 70% of all bacterial pneumonias • More common in men, elderly people, Blacks, and American Indians, in winter and early spring • Spread by air and contact with infectious secretions • Predisposing factors: trauma, viral infection, underlying pulmonary disease, overcrowded living quarters, chronic diseases, immunodeficiency • Among the 10 leading causes of death in the United States	• Sudden onset with severe shaking chills, temperature of 102° to 105° F (38.9° to 40.6° C), bacteremia, cough (with thick, scanty, blood-tinged sputum) accompanied by pleuritic pain • Malaise, weakness, and prostration common • Tachypnea, anorexia, nausea, and vomiting less common • Severity of pneumonia usually due to host's cellular defenses, not bacterial virulence
Otitis media • About 76% to 95% of all children have otitis media at least once. *S. pneumoniae* causes half of these cases.	• Ear pain, ear drainage, hearing loss, fever, lethargy, irritability • Other possible symptoms: vertigo, nystagmus, tinnitus
Meningitis • Can follow bacteremic pneumonia, mastoiditis, sinusitis, skull fracture, or endocarditis • Mortality (30% to 60%) highest in infants and in elderly people	• Fever, headache, nuchal rigidity, vomiting, photophobia, lethargy, coma

Bacteremia

Stemming possibly from a staphylococcal abscess or complicating recovery for patients with severe burns, bacteremia may be life-threatening. The prognosis is poor in patients over age 60 or in those with advanced cancer.

DIAGNOSIS	COMPLICATIONS	TREATMENT AND SPECIAL CONSIDERATIONS
• Isolation of group B streptococci from blood or infection site	• Bacteremia followed by meningitis or endocarditis	• Ampicillin or penicillin I.V. • Careful observation for symptoms of infection following delivery • Drainage and secretion precautions
• Gram stain of sputum shows gram-positive diplococci; culture shows *S. pneumoniae.* • Chest X-ray shows lobular consolidation in adults; bronchopneumonia in children and elderly people. • Elevated WBC count • Blood cultures often positive for *S. pneumoniae*	• Pleural effusion occurs in 25% of patients. • Pericarditis (rare) • Lung abscess (rare) • Death possible if bacteremia is present	• Penicillin or erythromycin I.V. or I.M. • Monitor and support respirations as needed. Record sputum color and amount. • Prevent dehydration. • Avoid sedatives and narcotics to preserve cough reflex. • Carefully dispose of all purulent drainage. (Respiratory isolation is unnecessary.) Advise high-risk patients to receive vaccine and to avoid infected persons.
• Fluid in middle ear • Isolation of *S. pneumoniae* from aspirated fluid if necessary	• Recurrent attacks may cause hearing loss.	• Amoxicillin or ampicillin • Tell patient to report lack of response to therapy after 72 hours.
• Isolation of *S. pneumoniae* from CSF or blood culture • Increased CSF cell count and protein level; decreased CSF glucose level	• Persistent hearing deficits, convulsions, hemiparesis, or other nerve deficits	• Penicillin I.V. or chloramphenicol • Monitor closely for neurologic changes. • Watch for symptoms of septic shock, such as acidosis and tissue hypoxia.

Causes   Bacteremia may result from infected surgical wounds, abscesses, infected I.V. or intra-arterial catheter sites or catheter tips, infected vascular grafts or prostheses, infected pressure ulcers, osteomyelitis, parenteral drug abuse, cellulitis, burns, immunosuppression, debilitating diseases (such as chronic renal insufficiency or diabetes), infective endocarditis (coagulase-positive staphylococci) and subacute infective endocarditis (coagulase-negative staphylococci), cancer (leukemia), or neutrophil nadir after chemotherapy or radiation, or the source may be unknown (primary bacteremia).

Signs and symptoms

The patient with developing bacteremia typically exhibits fever (with no obvious source in children under age 1), shaking chills, tachycardia, cyanosis or pallor, confusion, and agitation or stupor. In addition, he may have skin microabscesses from emboli-containing bacteria and joint pain.

Complications of bacteremia may include shock (likely in gram-negative bacteremia); acute infective endocarditis (indicated by new or changing systolic murmur in a prolonged infection); retinal hemorrhages (Roth's spots); splinter hemorrhages under the nails and small, tender red nodes on pads of fingers and toes (Osler's nodes); metastatic abscess formation in the skin, bones, lungs, brain, or kidneys; and pulmonary emboli if the tricuspid valve sustains infection.

Diagnosis

Common diagnostic findings in bactermia are:
• blood cultures (two to four samples from different sites at different times) that grow staphylococci
• leukocytosis (usually white blood cell count > 12,000/mm³), with shift to the left of polymorphonuclear leukocytes (70% to 90% neutrophils)
• urinalysis results showing hematuria
• elevated erythrocyte sedimentation rate, especially in chronic or subacute bacterial endocarditis
• blood test results indicating severe anemia and, possibly, thrombocytopenia; prolonged prothrombin time and partial thromboplastin time; low fibrinogen and platelet counts; low factor assays; and possibly disseminated intravascular coagulation.

Additional tests may include:
• cultures of urine, sputum, and draining skin lesions; chest X-rays; and scans of the lungs, liver, abdomen, and brain to identify the primary infection site
• an echocardiogram to detect bacterial vegetation on heart valves.

Treatment

Essential therapy includes antibiotics. Among drug choices are semisynthetic penicillins (oxacillin, nafcillin) or cephalosporins (cefazolin) given I.V; vancomycin also given I.V. for patients with a penicillin allergy or with methicillin-resistant infectious organisms; probenecid to partially prevent urinary excretion of penicillin and to prolong therapeutic levels of the drug; I.V. fluids to reverse shock; removal of an infected catheter or foreign body; and, possibly, surgery to excise the infection.

Special considerations

• Because bacteremia from *Staphylococcus aureus* can be fatal within 12 hours, be especially alert for it in debilitated patients with I.V. catheters or in those with a history of drug abuse.
• Administer antibiotics on time to maintain adequate blood levels. However, give them slowly, using the prescribed amount of diluent, to prevent thrombophlebitis.
• Watch for signs of penicillin allergy, especially pruritic rash (a sign of possible anaphylaxis). Keep epinephrine 1:1,000 and resuscitation equipment handy. Monitor vital signs, urine output, and mental state for signs of shock.
• Obtain specimens for culture carefully, and observe for clues to the primary site of infection. Never refrigerate blood culture specimens because refrigeration delays identification of organisms by slowing their growth.
• Impose wound and skin precautions if the primary site of infection is draining. Special blood precautions are not necessary because the number of organisms present, even in fulminant bacteremia, is minimal.
• Obtain peak and trough levels of vancomycin to determine the adequacy of treatment.

Staphylococcal pneumonia

An acute infection of the lung parenchyma, staphylococcal pneumonia typically impairs gas exchange and may involve the bronchial structures and the pulmonary lobes. The infection may be classified as primary, secondary, or aspiration pneumonia. Considered a primary pneumonia, this disease results from inhalation or aspiration of a staphylococcal pathogen. It occurs in both sexes and all age-groups. The prognosis is good for patients with normal lungs and adequate immune systems. In debilitated patients, bacterial pneumonia ranks as a leading cause of death. Complications of the disease include necrosis, lung abscess, pyopneumothorax, empyema, pneumatocele, shock, hypotension, oliguria or anuria, cyanosis, and loss of consciousness.

Causes

Factors that predispose a person to staphylococcal pneumonia—besides the infecting organism—include immune deficiencies, especially in elderly people and children under age 2; chronic lung diseases (such as cystic fibrosis); cancer; use of antibiotics that kill normal respiratory flora but spare *S. aureus;* and viral respiratory infections, especially influenza.

Other causes include hematogenous (blood-borne) bacteria spread to the lungs from primary sites of infections (such as heart valves, abscesses, and pulmonary emboli) and recent bronchial or endotracheal suctioning or intubation.

Signs and symptoms

Among characteristic signs and symptoms are a high temperature (103° to 105° F [39.4° to 40.6° C] in adults, 101° F [38.3° C] in children), cough with purulent yellow or bloody sputum, dyspnea, crackles, decreased breath sounds, and pleural pain.

In infants the disease may appear as a mild respiratory infection that suddenly worsens, as signaled by irritability, dyspnea, anorexia, vomiting, diarrhea, spasms of dry coughing, marked tachypnea, expiratory grunting, sternal retractions, and cyanosis.

Diagnosis

• White blood cell count: elevated (15,000 to 40,000/mm³ in adults; 15,000 to 20,000/mm³ in children), with predominance of polymorphonuclear leukocytes
• Sputum Gram stain: mostly gram-positive cocci in clusters, with many polymorphonuclear leukocytes
• Sputum culture: mostly coagulase-positive staphylococci
• Chest X-rays: usually patchy infiltrates
• Arterial blood gas analysis (in patients in shock): hypoxia and respiratory acidosis

Treatment

Therapeutic measures include antibiotic therapy with semi-synthetic penicillins (oxacillin, nafcillin) or cephalosporins given I.V., vancomycin given I.V. for those with penicillin allergy or methicillin-resistant organisms, and isolation until sputum shows minimal number of *S. aureus* (about 24 to 72 hours after starting antibiotic therapy).

Special considerations

• Use masks with patients in isolation because the staphylococci that infect the lungs are spread by air as well as by direct contact. Wear a gown and gloves when handling contaminated respiratory secretions.
• Keep the door to the patient's room closed. Don't store extra supplies in his room. Empty suction bottles carefully. Place any articles containing sputum (such as paper tissues or clothing) in a sealed plastic bag. Mark them "contaminated" and dispose of them promptly according to your hospital's policy.
• When obtaining sputum specimens, make sure that you're collecting thick sputum, not saliva. A specimen containing epithelial cells (found in the mouth, not the lungs) indicates a poor specimen.
• Administer antibiotics strictly on time, but slowly. Watch for signs of penicillin allergy and for signs of infection at I.V. sites. Change the I.V. site at least every third day or according to your hospital's policy.
• Perform frequent chest physical therapy. Do chest percussion and postural drainage after intermittent positive-pressure breathing treatments. Concentrate on consolidated areas (revealed by X-rays or auscultation).

Osteomyelitis

A pyogenic bone infection, osteomyelitis may be chronic or acute. The disease commonly follows traumatic injury—usually minor, but severe enough to cause a hematoma—and acute infection originating elsewhere in the body.

Typically a blood-borne disease, acute osteomyelitis most often affects the bones (especially the femur and tibia) of rapidly growing children, particularly boys under age 12. About 20% of affected children develop a chronic infection if not properly treated. The rarer chronic form of osteomyelitis is characterized by multiple draining sinus tracts and metastatic lesions. The incidence of both types of osteomyelitis is declining, except in drug abusers.

Causes

Bacterial and hematogenous organisms cause osteomyelitis. Factors that increase the risk for this disease include skin trauma, existing infection spread from adjacent joint or other infected tissues, *Staphylococcus aureus* bacteremia, orthopedic surgery or trauma, and cardiothoracic surgery.

Signs and symptoms

One of the first signs of osteomyelitis is the abrupt onset of fever—usually 101° F (38.3° C) or lower; shaking chills; pain and swelling over the infected area; restlessness; and headache.

Diagnosis

Besides the possible history of prior trauma to the involved area, the following test findings suggest osteomyelitis:
• positive bone and pus cultures (and blood cultures in about 50% of patients)
• X-ray changes apparent after the second or third week of the infection
• elevated erythrocyte sedimentation rate with a leukocyte shift to the left.

Treatment

Once osteomyelitis is identified, treatment consists of surgical debridement, prolonged antibiotic therapy (4 to 8 weeks), or vancomycin administered I.V. for those patients with penicillin allergy or methicillin-resistant organisms.

Special considerations

• After identifying the infected area, include it on the medical record.
• Check the penetration wound from which the organism originated for evidence of present infection.
• If severe pain renders the patient immobile, perform passive range-of-motion exercises. Apply heat as needed and elevate the affected part. (Extensive involvement may require casting until the infection subsides.)
• Before such procedures as surgical debridement, forewarn the patient to expect some pain. Explain that drainage is es-

sential for healing and that he will continue to receive analgesics and antibiotics after surgery.

Streptococcal pharyngitis

Commonly known as strep throat, streptococcal pharyngitis accounts for about 95% of all cases of bacterial pharyngitis. The infection is common in children ages 5 to 10 and occurs primarily from October to April.

Causes

The streptococcal organism that causes this infection is spread by direct person-to-person contact via droplets of saliva or nasal secretions. The streptococci frequently colonize in the throats of persons who exhibit no symptoms. Up to 20% of school children may be symptomless carriers.

Signs and symptoms

After a 1- to 5-day incubation period, initial signs and symptoms include a temperature of 101° to 104° F (38.3° to 40° C), a sore throat with severe pain on swallowing, beefy red pharynx, tonsillar exudate, edematous tonsils and uvula, swollen glands along the jaw line, generalized malaise and weakness, anorexia, and occasional abdominal discomfort.

Up to 40% of small children have symptoms too mild for diagnosis. Usually, the fever abates in 3 to 5 days, and nearly all symptoms subside within a week. Rarely, bacteremic spread may cause arthritis, endocarditis, meningitis, osteomyelitis, or liver abscess.

Diagnosis

Clinically indistinguishable from viral pharyngitis, bacterial pharyngitis may be detected by various tests, including:
• throat culture showing group A beta-hemolytic streptococci (carriers have positive throat culture)
• elevated white blood cell count
• serologic studies showing a fourfold rise in streptozyme titers during convalescence.

Treatment

The usual treatment for streptococcal pharyngitis is antibiotic therapy with penicillin or erythromycin.

Special considerations
• Stress the need for bed rest and isolation from others for 24 hours after antibiotic therapy begins.
• Instruct the patient to finish the full prescription and not to skip doses, even if the symptoms subside. Explain that abscess, glomerulonephritis, and rheumatic fever can occur with incomplete treatment.
• Teach the patient how to properly dispose of soiled paper tissues.

Impetigo

Also called streptococcal pyoderma, impetigo occurs most commonly in children ages 2 to 5 and in hot, humid weather. The disease has a high rate of spread (especially within families). Rarely, septicemia and ecthyma are complications of the infection.

Causes
The most common cause of impetigo is a streptococcal organism. Predisposing factors include close contact in schools, overcrowded living quarters, poor skin hygiene, and minor skin trauma. Transmission routes include direct contact, environmental contamination, and arthropod vectors.

Signs and symptoms
The appearance of small macules that rapidly develop into vesicles that become pustular and encrusted are the initial signs of impetigo. The progressing infection then causes pain, surrounding erythema, regional adenitis, cellulitis, and itching. Scratching spreads the infection.
    Lesions frequently affect the face, heal slowly, and leave depigmented areas.

Diagnosis
The differential diagnosis is usually made after observation of characteristic skin lesions having a honey-colored crust, then confirmed when a culture and Gram stain of swabbed lesions show *Streptococcus pyogenes*.

Treatment
The treatments of choice include penicillin given I.V. or orally, erythromycin, or antibiotic ointments accompanied by

frequent washing of the lesions with soap and water and thorough drying.

Special
considerations
• Isolate patients who have draining wounds.
• Provide ample patient education. Concentrate on preventive measures—especially good hygiene and proper wound care.

Infective endocarditis

An infection of the endocardium, heart valves, or a cardiac prosthesis, infective endocarditis is most common in elderly patients and in I.V. drug abusers. The disease can be acute (usually caused by staphylococci), but most cases are subacute (usually caused by *Streptococcus viridans*). Untreated, endocarditis is usually fatal, but with proper intervention, about 70% of patients recover. The prognosis is worse when endocarditis causes severe valvular damage—leading to insufficiency and left ventricular failure—or when it involves a prosthetic valve.

Causes
Group A nonhemolytic streptococci cause many cases of infective endocarditis. However, staphylococci, enterococci, and many other organisms (including *Neisseria gonorrhoeae, Pseudomonas, Salmonella, Streptobacillus, Serratia marcescens* and a host of others) can be the cause as well. The disease commonly follows bacteremia from an obvious source such as a wound infection, septic thrombophlebitis, open-heart surgery involving prosthetic valves, or skin, bone, and lung infections.

Signs and
symptoms
Weakness, fatigue, weight loss, fever, night sweats, anorexia, arthralgia, and splenomegaly are among the traditional signs and symptoms of endocarditis. Inspection findings may disclose petechiae, splinter hemorrhages under the nails, Osler's nodes, Roth's spots, Janeway's lesions, and clubbing of the fingers (in long-standing disease).

Auscultation may disclose a loud, regurgitant murmur. A murmur that changes suddenly or a new murmur that develops during fever is a classic physical sign of endocarditis. Additional signs and symptoms include splenomegaly (in long-standing disease) and dyspnea, tachycardia, bibasilar crackles, and neck vein distention.

In 12% to 35% of patients with subacute endocarditis, embolization from vegetating lesions or diseased valve tissue may produce findings characteristic of splenic, renal, cerebral, or pulmonary infarction or peripheral vascular occlusion.

Diagnosis

Among diagnostic findings positive for endocarditis are anemia, increased erythrocyte sedimentation rate and serum immunoglobulin levels, and a positive blood culture for group D streptococci.

Treatment

In endocarditis, antibiotic therapy depends on the infecting organism. For example, penicillin may be prescribed for *S. bovis* (nonenterococcal group D streptococci), and penicillin or ampicillin and an aminoglycoside may be prescribed for enterococcal group D streptococci.

Supportive treatment includes bed rest, aspirin for fever and achiness, and sufficient fluid intake. Corrective surgery may be undertaken as well for severe valvular damage.

Special considerations

• Stress the importance of bed rest, and assist the patient with bathing and toileting if necessary.
• Obtain a complete drug and allergy history before administering antibiotic therapy.
• Administer antibiotic therapy on time to maintain consistent and therapeutic drug levels in the blood.
• Assess cardiovascular status frequently and watch for signs of left ventricular failure, such as dyspnea, hypotension, tachycardia, tachypnea, crackles, neck vein distention, edema, and weight gain. Check for changes in cardiac rhythm or conduction.
• Administer oxygen and evaluate arterial blood gas values as needed to ensure adequate oxygenation.
• Watch for signs of embolization (hematuria, pleuritic chest pain, left upper quadrant pain, or paresis), a common occurrence during the first 3 months of treatment. Tell the pa-

tient to watch for and report these signs (which may indicate impending peripheral vascular occlusion or splenic, renal, cerebral, or pulmonary infarction).
• Monitor the patient's renal status (including blood urea nitrogen levels, creatinine clearance values, and urine output) to check for signs of renal emboli and drug toxicity.

GRAM-NEGATIVE COCCI

Most gram-negative organisms cause organ-specific disorders. *Neisseria meningitidis*, however, causes meningitis and meningococcemia, which can become systemic.

Meningococcal infections

Two major meningococcal infections (meningitis and meningococcemia) are caused by the gram-negative bacterium *Neisseria meningitidis*, which also causes primary pneumonia, purulent conjunctivitis, endocarditis, sinusitis, and genital infections. Meningococcemia occurs as simple bacteremia, fulminant meningococcemia and, rarely, chronic meningococcemia. It often accompanies meningitis. Meningococcal infections may occur sporadically or in epidemics; virulent infections may be fatal within hours.

Causes

Meningococcal infections occur most often among children (ages 6 months to 1 year) and men, usually military recruits, because of overcrowding.

N. meningitidis has seven serogroups (A, B, C, D, X, Y, Z); group A causes most epidemics. These bacteria are often present in upper respiratory flora. Transmission takes place through inhalation of an infected droplet from a carrier (an estimated 2% to 38% of the population). The bacteria then localize in the nasopharynx. Following an incubation period of approximately 3 or 4 days, they spread through the bloodstream to joints, skin, adrenal glands, lungs, and the central nervous system. The tissue damage that results (possibly due to the effects of bacterial exotoxins) produces symptoms and, in fulminant meningococcemia and meningococcal bacteremia, progresses to hemorrhage, thrombosis, and necrosis.

Signs and symptoms

Clinical features of meningococcal infection vary. Symptoms of meningococcal bacteremia include sudden spiking fever, headache, sore throat, cough, chills, myalgia (in back and legs), arthralgia, tachycardia, tachypnea, mild hypotension, and a petechial, nodular, or maculopapular rash.

In 10% to 20% of patients, this progresses to fulminant meningococcemia, with extreme prostration, enlargement of skin lesions, disseminated intravascular coagulation (DIC), and shock. Unless it is treated promptly, fulminant meningococcemia results in death from respiratory or heart failure in 6 to 24 hours.

Characteristics of the rare chronic form of meningococcemia include intermittent fever, maculopapular rash, joint pain, and enlarged spleen.

Diagnosis

Isolation of *N. meningitidis* through a positive blood culture, cerebrospinal fluid (CSF) culture, or lesion scraping confirms the diagnosis, except in nasopharyngeal infections because *N. meningitidis* is present as part of the normal nasopharyngeal flora.

Tests that support the diagnosis include counterimmunoelectrophoresis of CSF or blood, low white blood cell count and, in patients with skin or adrenal hemorrhages, decreased platelet count and clotting levels. Diagnostic evaluation must rule out Rocky Mountain spotted fever and vascular purpurae.

Treatment

As soon as meningococcal infection is suspected, treatment begins with large doses of aqueous penicillin G or ampicillin, which is sometimes combined with a cephalosporin (such as cefoxitin or moxalactam) or, for the patient who is allergic to penicillin, chloramphenicol I.V. Therapy may also include mannitol for cerebral edema, heparin I.V. for DIC, dopamine for shock, and digoxin and a diuretic if congestive heart failure develops.

Supportive measures include fluid and electrolyte maintenance, proper ventilation (patent airway and oxygen, if necessary), insertion of an arterial or central venous pressure (CVP) line to monitor cardiovascular status, and bed rest.

Chemoprophylaxis with rifampin or minocycline is useful for hospital workers in close contact with the patient; minocycline can also temporarily eradicate the infection in carriers.

Special considerations

• Give I.V. antibiotics to maintain blood and CSF drug levels.
• Enforce bed rest in early stages. Provide a dark, quiet, restful environment.
• Maintain adequate ventilation with oxygen or a ventilator, if necessary. Suction and turn the patient frequently.
• Keep accurate intake and output records to maintain proper fluid and electrolyte levels. Monitor blood pressure, pulse, arterial blood gases, and CVP.
• Watch for complications, such as DIC, arthritis, endocarditis, and pneumonia.
• If the patient is receiving chloramphenicol, monitor complete blood count.
• Check the patient's drug history for allergies before giving antibiotics.

Preventing transmission

• Impose respiratory isolation until the patient has received antibiotic therapy for 24 hours.
• Label all meningococcal specimens. Deliver them to the laboratory quickly because meningococci are very sensitive to changes in humidity and temperature.
• Report all meningococcal infections to local public health authorities.

GRAM-POSITIVE BACILLI

These bacilli produce a violet color, using a Gram stain. Examples of infections caused by gram-positive bacilli include diphtheria, listeriosis, tetanus, botulism, gas gangrene, actinomycosis, and nocardiosis.

Diphtheria

An acute, highly contagious toxin-mediated infection, diphtheria is caused by *Corynebacterium diphtheriae,* a gram-positive rod that usually infects the respiratory tract, primarily involving the tonsils, nasopharynx, and larynx. Currently, cutaneous, GI, and wound diphtheria are seen more frequently in the United States and are often caused by nontoxigenic strains. The urinary tract, conjunctivae, and ears are rarely involved.

Causes

Transmission usually occurs through intimate contact or by airborne respiratory droplets from apparently healthy carriers or convalescing patients, because many more people carry this disease than contract active infection. Diphtheria is more prevalent during the colder months because of closer interpersonal contact indoors, but it may be contracted at any time during the year.

Thanks to effective immunization, diphtheria is rare in many parts of the world, including the United States. Since 1972, there has been an increase in cutaneous diphtheria, especially in the Pacific Northwest and the Southwest, particularly in areas where crowding and poor sanitation conditions prevail. Most victims are children under age 15. Diphtheria's mortality rate is up to 10%.

Signs and
symptoms

Most infections go unrecognized, especially in partially immunized individuals. After an incubation period of less than a week, clinical cases of diphtheria characteristically show a thick, patchy, grayish green membrane over the mucous membranes of the pharynx, larynx, tonsils, soft palate, and nose; fever; sore throat; and a rasping cough, hoarseness, and other symptoms similar to croup.

Attempts to remove the membrane usually cause bleeding, which is highly characteristic of diphtheria. If this membrane causes airway obstruction (particularly likely in laryngeal diphtheria), symptoms include tachypnea; stridor; possible cyanosis; suprasternal retractions; and suffocation, if untreated. In cutaneous diphtheria, skin lesions resemble impetigo.

Complications of diphtheria include myocarditis, necrologic involvement (primarily affecting motor fibers but possibly also sensory neurons), renal involvement, and pulmonary involvement (bronchopneumonia) due to *C. diphtheriae* or other superinfectious organisms.

Diagnosis

Examination showing the characteristic membrane and throat culture, or culture of other suspect lesions growing *C. diphtheriae,* confirm this diagnosis. Treatment must begin based on clinical findings and not wait for confirmation by culture.

Treatment

Standard treatment includes diphtheria antitoxin administered I.M. or I.V.; antibiotics, such as penicillin or erythromycin, to eliminate the organisms from the upper respiratory tract and other sites and to terminate the carrier state; and measures to prevent complications.

Special
considerations

• To prevent spread of this disease, stress the need for strict isolation. Teach proper disposal of nasopharyngeal secretions. Maintain infection precautions until after two consecutive negative nasopharyngeal cultures—at least 1 week after drug therapy stops.

• Suggest that family members later receive diphtheria toxoid (usually given as combined diphtheria and tetanus toxoids or a combination including pertussis vaccine for children under age 6) if they haven't been immunized. Treatment of exposed individuals with antitoxin remains controversial.

• Administer drugs as needed. Although it is time-consuming and hazardous, desensitization should be attempted if tests are positive, because diphtheria antitoxin is the only *specific* treatment available. Because mortality increases in direct proportion to the delay in antitoxin administration, the antitoxin is given before laboratory confirmation of the diagnosis if sensitivity tests are negative.

• Before giving diphtheria antitoxin, which is made from horse serum, obtain eye and skin tests to determine sensitivity. After giving antitoxin or penicillin, be alert for anaphylaxis, and keep epinephrine 1:1,000 and resuscitative equipment handy. In patients who receive erythromycin, watch for thrombophlebitis.

• Monitor respirations carefully, especially in laryngeal diphtheria (usually, such patients are in a high-humidity or croup tent). Watch for signs of airway obstruction, and be ready to give immediate life support, including intubation and tracheotomy.

• Watch for signs of shock, which can develop suddenly.

• Obtain cultures.

• If neuritis develops, tell the patient it's usually transient. Be aware that peripheral neuritis may not develop until 2 to 3 months after onset of the illness.

• Be alert for signs of myocarditis, such as development of heart murmurs or electrocardiogram changes. Ventricular fibrillation is a common cause of sudden death in diphtheria patients.

• Assign a primary nurse to increase the effectiveness of isolation. Reassure the patient that isolation is temporary.

• Stress the need for childhood immunizations to all parents. Report all cases to local public health authorities.

Listeriosis

An infection caused by the weakly hemolytic, gram-positive bacillus *Listeria monocytogenes,* listeriosis occurs most often in fetuses, in neonates (during the first 3 weeks of life), and in older or immunosuppressed adults. The infected fetus is usually stillborn or is born prematurely, almost always with lethal listeriosis. This infection produces milder illness in pregnant women and varying degrees of illness in older and immunosuppressed patients; their prognoses depend on the severity of underlying illness.

Causes

The primary method of interpersonal transmission is neonatal infection *in utero* (through the placenta) or during passage through an infected birth canal. Other modes of transmission may include inhaling contaminated dust; drinking contaminated, unpasteurized milk; coming in contact with infected animals, contaminated sewage or mud, or soil contaminated with feces containing *L. monocytogenes;* and, possibly, interpersonal transmission.

Signs and symptoms

Contact with *L. monocytogenes* commonly causes a transient asymptomatic carrier state. But sometimes it produces bacteremia and a febrile, generalized illness. In a pregnant woman, especially during the third trimester, listeriosis causes a mild illness with malaise, chills, fever, and back pain. However, her fetus may suffer severe uterine infection, abortion, premature delivery, or stillbirth. Transplacental infection may also cause early neonatal death or granulomatosis infantiseptica, which produces organ abscesses in infants.

Infection with *L. monocytogenes* commonly causes meningitis, resulting in tense fontanels, irritability, lethargy, seizures, and coma in neonates, and low-grade fever and personality changes in adults. Fulminant manifestations with coma are rare.

Diagnosis

L. monocytogenes is identified by its diagnostic tumbling motility on a wet mount of the culture. Other supportive diagnostic results include positive culture of blood, spinal fluid, drainage from cervical or vaginal lesions, or lochia from a mother with an infected infant, but isolation of the organism from these specimens is often difficult. Listeriosis also causes monocytosis.

Treatment

The treatment of choice is ampicillin or penicillin I.V. for 3 to 6 weeks, possibly with gentamicin to increase its effectiveness. Alternative treatments include erythromycin, chloramphenicol, tetracycline, or co-trimoxazole.

Ampicillin and penicillin G are best for treating meningitis due to *L. monocytogenes* because they cross the blood-brain barrier more easily. Pregnant women require prompt, vigorous treatment to combat fetal infection.

Special considerations

• Deliver specimens to the laboratory promptly. Because very few organisms may be present, take at least 10 ml of spinal fluid for culture.

• Use secretion precautions until a series of cultures are negative. Be especially careful when handling lochia from an infected mother and secretions from her infant's eyes, nose, mouth, and rectum, including meconium.

• Evaluate neurologic status at least every 2 hours. In an infant, check fontanels for bulging. Maintain adequate I.V. fluid intake; measure intake and output accurately.

• If the patient has central nervous system depression and becomes apneic, provide respiratory assistance, monitor respirations, and obtain frequent arterial blood gas measurements.

• Provide adequate nutrition by total parenteral nutrition, nasogastric tube feedings, or a soft diet.

• Allow parents to see and, if possible, hold their infant in the intestive care unit. Be flexible about visiting privileges. Keep parents informed of the infant's status and prognosis at all times.

• Reassure an infected newborn's parents, who may feel guilty about their infant's illness.

• Educate pregnant women to avoid infective materials on farms where listeriosis is endemic among livestock.

Tetanus

An acute exotoxin-mediated infection, tetanus (lockjaw) is caused by the anaerobic, spore-forming, gram-positive bacillus *Clostridium tetani*. Usually, such infection is systemic; less often it's localized. Tetanus is fatal in up to 60% of unimmunized persons, usually within 10 days of onset. When symptoms develop within 3 days after exposure, the prognosis is poor.

Causes

Normally, transmission is through a puncture wound that is contaminated by soil, dust, or animal excretions containing *C. tetani* or by way of burns and minor wounds. After C. *tetani* enters the body, it causes local infection and tissue necrosis. It also produces toxins that then enter the bloodstream and lymphatic system and eventually spread to central nervous system tissue. Tetanus occurs worldwide, but it's more prevalent in agricultural regions and developing countries that lack mass immunization programs. It's one of the most common causes of neonatal deaths in developing countries, where infants of unimmunized mothers are delivered under unsterile conditions. In such infants, the unhealed umbilical cord is the portal of entry.

In the United States, about 75% of all tetanus cases occur between April and September.

Signs and symptoms

The incubation period varies from 3 to 4 weeks in mild tetanus to under 2 days in severe tetanus. When symptoms occur within 3 days after injury, death is more likely. If tetanus remains localized, signs of onset are spasm and increased muscle tone near the wound.

If tetanus is generalized (systemic), indications include marked muscle hypertonicity; hyperactive deep tendon reflexes; tachycardia; profuse sweating; low-grade fever; and painful, involuntary muscle contractions in:
• neck and facial muscles, especially cheek muscles, resulting in locked jaw (trismus) and a grotesque, grinning expression called *risus sardonicus*
• somatic muscles, resulting in arched-back rigidity (opisthotonos), and boardlike abdominal rigidity
• intermittent generalized spasms, lasting several minutes, which may possibly result in cyanosis and sudden death by asphyxiation.

Despite such pronounced neuromuscular symptoms, cerebral and sensory functions remain normal. Complications include atelectasis, pneumonia, pulmonary emboli, acute gastric ulcers, flexion contractures, and cardiac arrhythmias.

Neonatal tetanus is always generalized. The first clinical sign is difficulty in sucking, which usually appears 3 to 10 days after birth. It progresses to total inability to suck with excessive crying, irritability, and nuchal rigidity.

C. Davis

Diagnosis

Frequently, the diagnosis must rest on clinical features, and a history of trauma and no previous tetanus immunization. Blood cultures and tetanus antibody tests are often negative; only one-third of patients have a positive wound culture. Cerebrospinal fluid pressure may rise above normal. Accurate diagnosis also must rule out meningitis, rabies, phenothiazine or strychnine toxicity, and other conditions that mimic tetanus.

Treatment

Within 72 hours after a puncture wound, a patient with no previous history of tetanus immunization first requires tetanus immune globulin (TIG) or tetanus antitoxin to confer temporary protection. Next, he needs active immunization with tetanus toxoid. A patient who has not received tetanus immunization within 5 years needs a booster injection of tetanus toxoid. If tetanus develops despite immediate treatment, the patient will require airway maintenance and a muscle relaxant, such as diazepam, to decrease muscle rigidity and spasm. If muscle contractions aren't relieved by muscle relaxants, a neuromuscular blocker may be needed. The patient with tetanus needs high-dose antibiotics (penicillin administered I.V., if he's not allergic to it).

Special considerations

• When caring for the tetanus victim, thoroughly debride and clean the injury site with 3% hydrogen peroxide, and check the patient's immunization history. Record the cause of injury. If it's an animal bite, report the case to local public health authorities.
• Before giving penicillin and TIG, antitoxin, or toxoid, review the patient's history of allergies to immunizations or penicillin. If he has a history of allergies, keep epinephrine 1:1,000 and emergency airway equipment available.
• Stress the importance of maintaining active immunization with a booster dose of tetanus toxoid every 10 years.
• If tetanus develops, maintain an adequate airway and ventilation to prevent pneumonia and atelectasis. Suction as needed and watch for signs of respiratory distress. Keep emergency airway equipment on hand because the patient may require artificial ventilation or oxygen administration.
• Maintain an I.V. line for medications and emergency care if necessary.

• Monitor the patient's electrocardiogram frequently for arrhythmias. Accurately record intake and output, and check vital signs often.
• Turn the patient frequently to prevent pressure ulcers and pulmonary stasis.
• Because minimal external stimulation provokes muscle spasms, keep the patient's room dark and quiet. Warn visitors not to upset or overstimulate the patient.
• If urine retention develops, insert an indwelling catheter.
• Give muscle relaxants and sedatives and schedule patient care, such as passive range-of-motion exercises, to coincide with periods of heaviest sedation.
• Insert an artificial airway, if necessary, to prevent tongue injury and maintain an airway during spasms.
• Provide adequate nutrition to meet the patient's increased metabolic needs. The patient may need nasogastric feedings or total parenteral nutrition.

Botulism

A life-threatening paralytic illness, botulism results from an exotoxin produced by the gram-positive, anaerobic bacillus *Clostridium botulinum.* It occurs with botulism food poisoning, wound botulism, and infant botulism. The mortality from botulism is about 25%, with death most often caused by respiratory failure during the first week of illness.

Causes

Botulism usually occurs as a result of ingesting inadequately cooked, contaminated foods, especially those with low acid content, such as home-canned fruits and vegetables, sausages, and smoked or preserved fish or meat. Rarely, it may result from wound infection with *C. botulinum.*

Botulism occurs worldwide and affects adults more often than children. Recent findings have shown that an infant's GI tract can become colonized with *C. botulinum* from some unknown source, and then the exotoxin is produced within the infant's intestine. Incidence had been declining, but the current trend toward home canning has resulted in an upswing of this disease (approximately 250 cases per year in the United States) in recent years.

Signs and symptoms

Most patients experience symptoms within 12 to 36 hours after ingesting contaminated food, but symptoms may appear as soon as 6 hours or up to 8 days after this time. Severity varies with the amount of toxin ingested and the patient's degree of immunocompetence. Generally, early onset (within 24 hours) of symptoms signals critical and potentially fatal illness. Initial symptoms include dry mouth, sore throat, weakness, vomiting, and diarrhea.

The cardinal symptom of botulism, though, is acute symmetrical cranial nerve impairment (ptosis, diplopia, dysarthria), followed by descending weakness or paralysis of muscles in the extremities or trunk, and dyspnea from respiratory muscle paralysis. Such impairment doesn't affect mental or sensory processes and isn't associated with fever.

Infant botulism typically occurs between 3 and 20 weeks of age and can produce hypotonic (floppy) infant syndrome. Symptoms are constipation, feeble cry, depressed gag reflex, and inability to suck. Cranial nerve deficits also occur in infants and are manifested by a flaccid facial expression, ptosis, and ophthalmoplegia. Infants also develop generalized muscle weakness, hypotonia, and areflexia. Loss of head control may be striking. Respiratory arrest is likely.

Diagnosis

Identification of the offending toxin in the patient's serum, stool, gastric contents, or the suspected food confirms the diagnosis. An electromyogram showing diminished muscle action potential after a single supramaximal nerve stimulus is also diagnostic.

Diagnosis also must rule out other diseases often confused with botulism, such as Guillain-Barré syndrome, myasthenia gravis, cerebrovascular accident, staphylococcal food poisoning, tick paralysis, chemical intoxications, carbon monoxide poisoning, fish poisoning, trichinosis, and diphtheria.

Treatment

If clinical signs of botulism appear, admit the patient to the intensive care unit, and monitor cardiac and respiratory function carefully. If ingestion has occurred within several hours, induce vomiting, begin gastric lavage, and give a high enema to purge any unabsorbed toxin from the bowel. Administer botulinum antitoxin I.V. or I.M. to neutralize any circulating toxin. (Botulinum antitoxin is available through the Centers for Disease Control and Prevention.) Before giving antitoxin, obtain an accurate patient history of allergies, especially to horses, and perform a skin test. Afterward, watch for anaphylaxis or other hypersensitivity reactions and serum sickness. Keep epinephrine 1:1,000 (for S.C. administration) and emergency airway equipment available.

Special considerations

• If you suspect ingestion of contaminated food, obtain a careful history of the patient's food intake for the past several days. Check to see if other family members exhibit similar symptoms and share a common food history.

• Observe carefully for abnormal neurologic signs. If the patient returns home, tell his family to watch for signs of weakness, blurred vision, and slurred speech, and to return the patient to the hospital immediately if such signs appear.

• Assess respiratory function every 4 hours. Be alert for decreased vital capacity on inspiratory effort and any signs of respiratory distress.

• Assess and record neurologic function, including bilateral motor status (reflexes, ability to move arms and legs).

• Give I.V. fluids as appropriate. Turn the patient often, and frequently encourage deep-breathing exercises. Isolation is not required.

• Because botulism is sometimes fatal, keep the patient and family informed regarding the course of the disease.

• Immediately report all cases of botulism to local public health authorities.

• To help prevent botulism, encourage safe processing and preserving of foods.

• Warn against even *tasting* food from a bulging can or one with a peculiar odor, and urge sterilizing any utensil that contacts suspected food; ingestion of even a small amount of food contaminated with botulism toxin can prove fatal.

Gas gangrene

A rare infection, gas gangrene results from local infection with the anaerobic, spore-forming, gram-positive rod *Clostridium perfringens* (or another clostridial species). It occurs in devitalized tissues and results from compromised arterial circulation following trauma or surgery.

Gas gangrene carries a high mortality unless therapy begins immediately. However, with prompt treatment, 80% of patients with gas gangrene of the extremities survive; prognosis is poorer for gas gangrene in other sites, such as the abdominal wall or the bowel. The usual incubation period is 1 to 4 days but can vary from 3 hours to 6 weeks or longer.

Causes

C. perfringens is a normal inhabitant of the GI and female genital tracts; it's also prevalent in soil. Transmission occurs by entry of organisms during trauma or surgery.

Because *C. perfringens* is anaerobic, gas gangrene is most often found in deep wounds, especially those in which tissue necrosis further reduces oxygen supply. When *C. perfringens* invades soft tissues, it produces thrombosis of regional blood vessels, tissue necrosis, and localized edema. Such necrosis releases both carbon dioxide and hydrogen subcutaneously, producing interstitial gas bubbles. Gas gangrene most commonly occurs in the extremities and in abdominal wounds, and less frequently in the uterus. (See *Growth cycle of* Clostridium perfringens.)

Signs and Symptoms

True gas gangrene produces myositis and another form of this disease, involving only soft tissue, called anaerobic cellulitis. Most signs of infection develop within 72 hours of trauma or surgery. The hallmark of gas gangrene is crepitation, a result of carbon dioxide and hydrogen accumulation as a metabolic by-product in necrotic tissues.

Other typical indications are severe localized pain, swelling, and discoloration (often dusky brown or reddish), with formation of bullae and necrosis within 36 hours from onset of symptoms. Soon the skin over the wound may rupture, revealing dark red or black necrotic muscle, a foul-smelling watery or frothy discharge, intravascular hemolysis,

Growth cycle of *Clostridium perfringens* (in a closed wound)

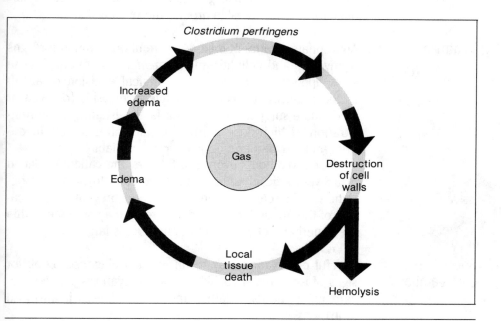

thrombosis of blood vessels, and evidence of infection spread.

In addition to these local symptoms, gas gangrene produces early signs of toxemia and hypovolemia (tachycardia, tachypnea, and hypotension), with moderate fever usually not above 101° F (38.3° C). Although pale, prostrate, and motionless, most patients remain alert and oriented and are extremely apprehensive. Usually death occurs suddenly, often during surgery for removal of necrotic tissue. Less often, death is preceded by delirium and coma and is sometimes accompanied by vomiting, profuse diarrhea, and circulatory collapse.

Diagnosis

A history of recent surgery or a deep puncture wound and the rapid onset of pain and crepitation around the wound suggest this diagnosis. It is confirmed by anaerobic cultures of wound drainage showing *C. perfringens;* a Gram stain of wound drainage showing large, gram-positive, rod-shaped bacteria; X-rays showing gas in tissues; and blood studies showing leukocytosis and, later, hemolysis.

Diagnosis must rule out synergistic gangrene and necrotizing fasciitis; unlike gas gangrene, both of these disorders anesthetize the skin around the wound.

Treatment

Appropriate treatment includes careful observation for signs of myositis and cellulitis and *immediate* treatment if these signs appear; *immediate* wide surgical excision of all affected tissues and necrotic muscle in myositis (delayed or inadequate surgical excision is a fatal mistake); I.V. administration of high-dose penicillin; and, after adequate debridement, hyperbaric oxygenation if available.

For 1 to 3 hours every 6 to 8 hours, the patient is placed in a hyperbaric chamber and is exposed to pressures designed to increase oxygen tension and prevent multiplication of the anaerobic clostridia. Surgery may be done within the hyperbaric chamber if the chamber is large enough.

Special considerations

Careful observation may result in early diagnosis. Look for signs of ischemia (cool skin; pallor or cyanosis; sudden, severe pain; sudden edema; and loss of pulses in involved limb).

• Throughout this illness, provide adequate fluid replacement, and assess pulmonary and cardiac functions often. Maintain airway and ventilation.

• To prevent skin breakdown and further infection, give good skin care. After surgery, provide meticulous wound care.

• Before penicillin administration, obtain a patient history of allergies; afterward, watch closely for signs of a hypersensitivity reaction.

• Psychological support is critical because patients with gas gangrene can remain alert until death, knowing that death is imminent and unavoidable.

• Deodorize the room to control foul odor from wound. Prepare the patient emotionally for a large wound after surgical excision, and refer him for physical rehabilitation as necessary.

• Institute wound precautions. Dispose of drainage material properly (double-bag dressings in plastic bags for incineration), and wear sterile gloves when changing dressings. No

special cleaning measures are required after the patient is discharged.
• To prevent gas gangrene, routinely take precautions to render all wound sites unsuitable for growth of clostridia by attempting to keep granulation tissue viable; adequate debridement is imperative to reduce anaerobic growth conditions.
• Be alert for devitalized tissues, and notify the surgeon promptly if you detect them. Position the patient to facilitate drainage, and eliminate all dead spaces in closed wounds.

Actinomycosis

The infection actinomycosis is primarily caused by the gram-positive anaerobic bacillus *Actinomyces israelii,* which produces granulomatous, suppurative lesions with abscesses. Common infection sites are the head, neck, thorax, and abdomen, but it can spread to contiguous tissues, causing multiple draining sinuses.

Sporadic and infrequent, actinomycosis affects twice as many males—usually ages 15 to 35—as females. It is likely in people with dental disease or human immunodeficiency virus infection.

Causes

A. israelii occurs as part of the normal flora of the throat, tonsillar crypts, and mouth (particularly around carious teeth); infection results from its traumatic introduction into body tissues.

Signs and symptoms

Symptoms appear from days to months after injury and may vary depending on the site of infection.

In cervicofacial actinomycosis (lumpy jaw), painful, indurated swellings appear in the mouth or neck up to several weeks following dental extraction or trauma. They gradually enlarge and form fistulae that open onto the skin. Sulfur granules (yellowish gray masses that are actually colonies of *A. israelii*) appear in the exudate.

In pulmonary actinomycosis, aspiration of bacteria from the mouth into areas of the lungs already anaerobic from infection or atelectasis produces a fever and a cough that becomes productive and occasionally causes hemoptysis. Eventually, empyema follows, a sinus forms through the chest wall, and septicemia may occur.

In GI actinomycosis, ileocecal lesions are caused by swallowed bacteria, which produce abdominal discomfort, fever, sometimes a palpable mass, and an external sinus. This follows intestinal mucosal disruption, usually by surgery or an inflammatory bowel condition such as appendicitis.

Rare sites of actinomycotic infection are the bones, brain, liver, kidneys, and female reproductive organs. Symptoms reflect the organ involved.

Diagnosis

Isolation of *A. israelii* in exudate or tissue confirms actinomycosis. Other tests that help identify it are:
• microscopic examination of sulfur granules
• Gram staining of excised tissue or exudate to reveal branching gram-positive rods
• chest X-ray to show lesions in unusual locations, such as the shaft of a rib.

Treatment

High-dose I.V. penicillin or tetracycline therapy precedes surgical excision and drainage of abscesses in all forms of the disease and continues for 3 to 6 weeks. Following parenteral therapy, treatment with oral penicillin or tetracycline may continue for 1 to 6 months.

Special considerations

• Dispose of all dressings in a sealed plastic bag.
• After surgery, provide proper aseptic wound management.
• Administer antibiotics. Before giving the first dose, obtain an accurate patient history of allergies. Watch for hypersensitivity reactions, such as rash, fever, itching, and signs of anaphylaxis. If the patient has a history of any allergies, keep epinephrine 1:1,000 and resuscitative equipment available.
• Stress the importance of good oral hygiene and proper dental care.

Nocardiosis

An acute, subacute, or chronic bacterial infection, nocardiosis is caused by a weakly gram-positive species of the genus *Nocardia* — usually *Nocardia asteroides*. It's most common in men, especially those with compromised immune defense mechanisms. Its mortality in brain infection exceeds 80%; in other forms, the mortality is 50% even with appropriate therapy.

Causes

Nocardia is a genus of aerobic, gram-positive bacteria with branching filaments similar in appearance to fungi. Normally found in soil, these organisms occasionally cause sporadic disease in humans and animals throughout the world. Their incubation period is unknown but is probably several weeks. The usual mode of transmission is inhalation of organisms suspended in dust; less often it's direct inoculation through puncture wounds or abrasions.

Signs and
symptoms

Nocardiosis originates as a pulmonary infection and causes a cough that produces thick, tenacious, purulent, mucopurulent, and possibly blood-tinged sputum. It may also cause a fever as high as 105° F (40.6° C), chills, night sweats, anorexia, malaise, and weight loss. This infection may lead to pleurisy, intrapleural effusion, empyema, tracheitis, bronchitis, pericarditis, endocarditis, peritonitis, mediastinitis, septic arthritis, and keratoconjunctivitis.

If the infection spreads through the blood to the brain, abscesses form, causing confusion, disorientation, dizziness, headache, nausea, and seizures. Rupture of a brain abscess can cause purulent meningitis. Extrapulmonary, hematogenous spread may cause endocarditis and lesions of kidneys, liver, subcutaneous tissue, and bone.

Diagnosis

Identification of *Nocardia* by culture of sputum or discharge is difficult. Special staining techniques often must be relied upon to make the diagnosis, in conjunction with a typical clinical picture (usually progressive pneumonia, despite antibiotic therapy). Occasionally, diagnosis requires biopsy of lung or other tissue. Chest X-rays vary and may show puffy or interstitial infiltrates, nodules, or abscesses. Unfortunately, up to 40% of nocardial infections elude diagnosis until postmortem examination.

In brain infection with meningitis, lumbar puncture shows nonspecific changes, such as increased pressure at the opening; cerebrospinal fluid shows in white blood cell and protein levels, and decreased glucose levels compared to serum glucose.

Treatment

Nocardiosis requires 12 to 18 months of treatment, preferably with co-trimoxazole or high doses of sulfonamides. In patients who do not respond to sulfonamide treatment, other drugs, such as ampicillin or erythromycin, may be added. Treatment also includes surgical drainage of abscesses and excision of necrotic tissue. The acute phase requires complete bed rest; as the patient improves, activity can increase.

Special considerations

• Nocardiosis requires no isolation: it's not transmitted from person to person.
• Provide adequate nourishment through total parenteral nutrition, nasogastric tube feedings, or a balanced diet.
• Give tepid sponge baths and antipyretics to reduce fever.
• Monitor for allergic reactions to antibiotics.
• High-dose sulfonamide therapy (especially sulfadiazine) predisposes the patient to crystalluria and oliguria. So assess him frequently, force fluids, and alkalinize the urine with sodium bicarbonate to prevent these complications.
• In patients with pulmonary infection, administer chest physiotherapy. Auscultate the lungs daily, checking for increased crackles or consolidation. Note and record amount, color, and thickness of sputum.
• In brain infection, regularly assess neurologic function. Watch for signs of increased intracranial pressure, such as decreased level of consciousness, and respiratory abnormalities.
• In long-term hospitalization, turn the patient often, and assist with range-of-motion exercises.
• Before the patient is discharged, stress the need for a regular medication schedule to maintain therapeutic blood levels and continuation of drugs even after symptoms subside.
• Explain the importance of frequent follow-up examinations.

• Provide support and encouragement to help the patient and his family cope with this long-term illness.

GRAM-NEGATIVE BACILLI

Infections caused by gram-negative bacilli may be mild to life-threatening and may have local or systemic effects. Such infections include *Salmonella* infection, shigellosis, *Escherichia coli* and other Enterobacteriaceae infections, *Pseudomonas* infections, and many others.

Salmonellosis

A common infection in the United States, salmonellosis is caused by gram-negative bacilli of the genus *Salmonella*, a member of the Enterobacteriaceae family. (See *Incidence of salmonellosis in the United States*, page 54.) It occurs as enterocolitis, bacteremia, localized infection, typhoid, or paratyphoid fever. Nontyphoidal forms usually produce mild to moderate illness with low mortality.

Typhoid, the most severe form of salmonellosis, usually lasts from 1 to 4 weeks. About 3% of persons who are treated and 10% of those who are untreated die, usually as a result of intestinal perforation or hemorrhage, cerebral thrombosis, toxemia, pneumonia, or acute circulatory failure. An attack of typhoid confers lifelong immunity, although the patient may become a carrier.

Salmonellosis occurs 20 times more often in patients with acquired immunodeficiency syndrome. Specific features are increased incidence of bacteremia, inability to identify the infection's source, and tendency of the infection to recur after therapy is stopped. Therefore, long-term suppressive drug therapy may be needed.

Incidence of salmonellosis in the United States

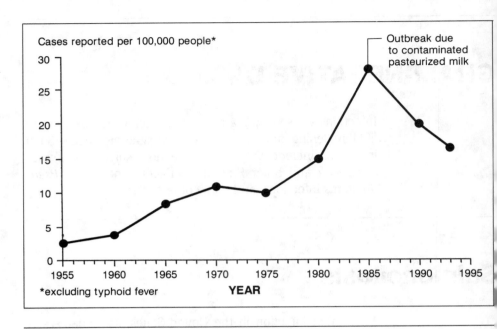

Cases reported per 100,000 people*

Outbreak due to contaminated pasteurized milk

*excluding typhoid fever

YEAR

Causes

Of an estimated 1,700 serotypes of *Salmonella,* 10 cause the diseases most common in the United States; all 10 can survive for weeks in water, ice, sewage, or food. Nontyphoidal salmonellosis generally follows the ingestion of contaminated or inadequately processed foods, especially eggs, chicken, turkey, and duck. Proper cooking reduces the risk of contracting salmonellosis. Other causes include contact with infected persons or animals or ingestion of contaminated dry milk, chocolate bars, or pharmaceuticals of animal origin. Salmonellosis may occur in children under age 5 from fecal-oral spread. Enterocolitis and bacteremia are common among infants, elderly people, and people already weakened by other infections; paratyphoid fever is rare in the United States.

Typhoid results most frequently from drinking water contaminated by excretions of a carrier. Most typhoid patients are under age 30; most carriers are women over age 50. Incidence of typhoid in the United States is increasing as a result of travelers returning from endemic areas.

Clinical variants of salmonellosis

VARIANT	CAUSE	CLINICAL FEATURES
Enterocoli-tis	Any species of nontyphoidal *Salmonella,* but usually *S. enteritidis.* Incubation period is 6 to 48 hours.	• Mild to severe abdominal pain, diarrhea, sudden fever to 102° F (38.9° C), nausea, vomiting • Usually self-limiting, but may progress to enteric fever (resembling typhoid), local abscesses (usually abdominal), dehydration, septicemia
Paratyphoid	*S. paratyphi* and *S. schottmuelleri* (formerly *S. paratyphi B*). Incubation period is 3 weeks or more.	• Fever and transient diarrhea • Generally resembles typhoid but less severe
Bacteremia	Any *Salmonella* species, but most commonly *S. choleraesuis.* Incubation period varies.	• Fever, chills, anorexia, weight loss (without GI symptoms), joint pain
Localized infections	Usually follows bacteremia caused by *Salmonella* species.	• Site of localization determines symptoms. • Localized abscesses may cause osteomyelitis, endocarditis, bronchopneumonia, pyelonephritis, and arthritis.
Typhoid fever	*S. typhi* enters GI tract and invades the bloodstream via the lymphatics, setting up intracellular sites. During this phase, infection of biliary tract leads to intestinal seeding with millions of bacilli. Involved lymphoid tissues (especially Peyer's patches in ilium) enlarge, ulcerate, and necrose, resulting in hemorrhage. Incubation period is usually 1 to 2 weeks.	Symptoms of enterocolitis may develop within hours of ingesting *S. typhi;* they usually subside before onset of typhoid fever symptoms. • *First week:* gradually increasing fever, anorexia, myalgia, malaise, headache • *Second week:* remittent fever up to 104° F (40° C) usually in the evening, chills, diaphoresis, weakness, delirium, increasing abdominal pain and distention, diarrhea or constipation, cough, moist crackles, tender abdomen with enlarged spleen, maculopapular rash (especially on abdomen) • *Third week:* persistent fever, increasing fatigue and weakness; usually subsides by end of third week, although relapses may occur • *Complications:* intestinal perforation or hemorrhage, abscesses, thrombophlebitis, cerebral thrombosis, pneumonia, osteomyelitis, myocarditis, acute circulatory failure, chronic carrier state

Signs and symptoms

Clinical manifestations of salmonellosis vary but usually include fever, abdominal pain, and severe diarrhea with enterocolitis. Headache, increasing fever, and constipation are more common with typhoidal infection. (See *Clinical variants of salmonellosis.*)

Diagnosis

Generally, positive diagnosis depends on isolation of the organism in a culture, particularly blood (in typhoid, paratyphoid, and bacteremia) or feces (in enterocolitis, paratyphoid, and typhoid). Other appropriate culture specimens include urine, bone marrow, pus, and vomitus. In endemic areas, clinical symptoms of enterocolitis allow a working diagnosis before the cultures are positive. Presence of *S. typhi* in stools 1 or more years after treatment indicates that the patient is a carrier, which is true of 3% of patients.

Widal's test, an agglutination reaction against somatic and flagellar antigens, may suggest typhoid with a fourfold rise in titer. However, drug use or hepatic disease can also increase these titers and invalidate test results. Other supportive laboratory values may include transient leukocytosis during the first week of typhoidal salmonellosis, leukopenia during the third week, and leukocytosis in local infection.

Treatment

Antimicrobial therapy for typhoid, paratyphoid, and bacteremia depends on organism sensitivity. It may include amoxicillin, chloramphenicol and, in severely toxemic patients, cotrimoxazole, ciprofloxacin, or ceftriaxone. Localized abscesses may also need surgical drainage. Enterocolitis requires a short course of antibiotics only if it causes septicemia or prolonged fever.

Symptomatic treatment includes bed rest and replacement of fluids and electrolytes. Camphorated opium tincture, kaolin with pectin, diphenoxylate hydrochloride, codeine, or small doses of morphine may relieve diarrhea and control cramps in patients who must remain active.

Special considerations

• Follow enteric precautions. Always wash your hands thoroughly before and after any contact with the patient, and advise other hospital personnel to do the same. Teach the patient to use proper hand-washing technique, especially after defecating and before eating or handling food. Wear gloves and a gown when disposing of feces or fecally contaminated objects.

• Continue enteric precautions until results of three consecutive stool cultures are negative—the first one 48 hours after antibiotic treatment ends, followed by two more at 24-hour intervals.

• Observe the patient closely for signs of bowel perforation: sudden pain in the right lower abdominal quadrant, possibly after one or more rectal bleeding episodes; sudden fall in temperature or blood pressure; and rising pulse rate.

• During acute infection, plan your care and other activities to allow the patient as much rest as possible. Raise the side rails and use other safety measures because the patient may become delirious. Assign him a room close to the nurses' station so he can be checked on often.

• Use a room deodorizer (preferably electric) to minimize odor from diarrhea and to provide a comfortable atmosphere for rest.

• Accurately record intake and output. Maintain adequate I.V. hydration. When the patient can tolerate oral feedings, encourage high-calorie fluids such as milk shakes. Watch for constipation.

• Provide good skin and mouth care. Turn the patient frequently, and perform range-of-motion exercises as indicated. Apply mild heat to the abdomen to relieve cramps.

• *Don't* administer antipyretics. These mask fever and lead to possible hypothermia. Instead, to promote heat loss through the skin without causing shivering (which keeps fever high by vasoconstriction), apply tepid, wet towels (don't use alcohol or ice) to the patient's groin and axillae.

• To promote heat loss by vasodilation of peripheral blood vessels, use additional wet towels on the arms and legs, wiping with long, vigorous strokes.

• After draining the abscesses of a joint, provide heat, elevation, and passive range-of-motion exercises to decrease swelling and maintain mobility.

• If the patient has positive stool cultures on discharge, tell him to use a different bathroom than other family members if possible (while he's on antibiotics); to wash his hands afterward; and to avoid preparing uncooked foods, such as salads, for family members.

• To prevent salmonellosis, advise prompt refrigeration of meat and cooked foods (avoid keeping them at room temperature for any prolonged period), and teach the importance of proper hand washing. Advise those at high risk for contracting typhoid (laboratory workers, travelers) to seek vaccination.

Shigellosis

An acute intestinal infection, shigellosis (bacillary dysentery) is caused by the bacterium *Shigella,* a short, nonmotile, gram-negative rod. *Shigella* can be classified into four groups, all of which may cause shigellosis: group A *(Shigella dysenteriae),* which is most common in Central America and causes particularly severe infection and septicemia; group B *(Shigella flexneri);* group C *(Shigella boydii);* and group D *(Shigella sonnei).* Typically, shigellosis causes a high fever (especially in children); acute, self-limiting diarrhea with tenesmus (ineffectual straining to defecate); and possibly electrolyte imbalance and dehydration.

Shigellosis is most common in children ages 1 to 4, but adults often acquire it from children. The prognosis is good. Mild infections usually subside within 10 days; severe infections may persist for 2 to 6 weeks. With prompt treatment, shigellosis is fatal in only 1% of cases; however, in severe *Shigella dysenteriae* epidemics, mortality may reach 8%.

Causes

Shigellosis is endemic in North America, Europe, and the tropics. In the United States, about 23,000 cases appear annually, usually in children or in elderly, debilitated, or malnourished people. Shigellosis commonly occurs among confined populations, such as those in mental institutions or hospitals. In Great Britain, its incidence is rising, despite improved sanitation and infection control.

Transmission is through the fecal-oral route, by direct contact with contaminated objects, or through ingestion of contaminated food or water. Occasionally, the housefly is a vector.

Signs and symptoms

After an incubation period of 1 to 4 days, *Shigella* organisms invade the intestinal mucosa and cause inflammation. In children, shigellosis usually produces high fever, diarrhea with tenesmus, nausea, vomiting, irritability, drowsiness, and abdominal pain and distention. Within a few days, the child's stool may contain pus, mucus, and — from the superficial intestinal ulceration typical of this infection — blood. Without treatment, dehydration and weight loss are rapid and overwhelming.

In adults, shigellosis produces sporadic, intense abdominal pain, which may be relieved at first by passing formed stools. Eventually, however, it causes rectal irritability, tenesmus and, in severe infection, headache and prostration. Stools may contain pus, mucus, and blood. In adults, shigellosis doesn't usually cause fever.

Complications of shigellosis are not common but may be fatal in children and debilitated patients and include electrolyte imbalance (especially hypokalemia), metabolic acidosis, and shock. Less common complications include conjunctivitis, iritis, arthritis, rectal prolapse, secondary bacterial infection, acute blood loss from mucosal ulcers, and toxic neuritis.

Diagnosis

Fever (in children) and diarrhea with stools containing blood, pus, and mucus point to this diagnosis; microscopic bacteriologic studies and culture help confirm it. Microscopic examination of a fresh stool may reveal mucus, red blood cells, and polymorphonuclear leukocytes; direct immunofluorescence with specific antisera may reveal *Shigella*. Severe infection increases hemagglutinating antibodies. Sigmoidoscopy or proctoscopy may reveal typical superficial ulcerations.

Diagnosis must rule out other causes of diarrhea, such as enteropathogenic *Escherichia coli* infection, malabsorption disorders, and amoebic or viral diseases.

Treatment

Appropriate treatment of shigellosis includes enteric precautions, low-residue diet, and most importantly, replacement of fluids and electrolytes with I.V. infusions of 0.9% sodium chloride solution (with electrolytes) in sufficient quantities to maintain a urine output of 40 to 50 ml/hour.

Antibiotics are of questionable value but may be used in an attempt to eliminate the pathogen and thereby prevent further spread. Ampicillin, tetracycline, or co-trimoxazole may be useful in severe cases, especially in children with overwhelming fluid and electrolyte losses. Antidiarrheals that slow intestinal motility are contraindicated in shigellosis, because they delay fecal excretion of *Shigella* and prolong fever and diarrhea. An investigational vaccine containing attenuated strains of *Shigella* appears promising in preventing shigellosis.

Special considerations

• To prevent dehydration, administer I.V. fluids. Measure intake and output (including stools) carefully.
• Correct identification of *Shigella* requires examination and culture of a fresh stool specimen. Therefore, hand-carry specimens directly to the laboratory. Because shigellosis is suspected, include this information on the laboratory slip.
• Use a disposable hot-water bottle to relieve abdominal discomfort, and schedule care to conserve patient strength.
• To help prevent spread of this disease, maintain enteric precautions until microscopic bacteriologic studies confirm that the stool specimen is negative. If a risk of exposure to the patient's stools exists, put on a gown and gloves before entering the room.
• Keep the patient's (and your own) nails short to avoid harboring organisms. Change soiled linens promptly and store them in an isolation container.
• During shigellosis outbreaks, obtain stool specimens from all potentially infected staff, and instruct those infected to remain away from work until two stool specimens are negative.

Escherichia coli and other Enterobacteriaceae infections

Enterobacteriaceae—a family of mostly aerobic, gram-negative bacilli—causes local and systemic infections, including an invasive diarrhea resembling shigella and, more often, a noninvasive toxin-mediated diarrhea resembling cholera. This group of bacteria, including *Escherichia coli,* causes most nosocomial infections. Noninvasive, enterotoxin-producing *E. coli* infections may be a major cause of diarrheal illness in children in the United States.

The prognosis in cases of mild to moderate infection is good. But severe infection requires immediate fluid and electrolyte replacement to avoid fatal dehydration, espe-

Enterobacteriaceae infections

The Enterobacteriaceae include *Escherichia coli, Arizona, Citrobacter, Enterobacter, Erwinia, Hafnia, Klebsiella, Morganella, Proteus, Providencia, Salmonella, Serratia, Shigella,* and *Yersinia.*

Exogenous or endogenous
Enterobacterial infections are exogenous (from other people or the environment), endogenous (from one part of the body to another), or a combination of both. Enterobacteriaceae infections may cause any of a long list of bacterial diseases: bacterial (gram-negative) pneumonia, empyema, endocarditis, osteomyelitis, septic arthritis, urethritis, cystitis, bacterial prostatitis, urinary tract infection, pyelonephritis, perinephric abscess, abdominal abscesses, cellulitis, skin ulcers, appendicitis, gastroenterocolitis, diverticulitis, eyelid and periorbital cellulitis, corneal conjunctivitis, meningitis, bacteremia, and intracranial abscesses.

Treatment
Appropriate antibiotic therapy depends on the results of culture and sensitivity tests. Generally, the aminoglycosides, cephalosporins, and penicillins—such as ampicillin, mezlocillin, and piperacillin—are most effective.

---

cially among children, in whom mortality may be quite high. (See *Enterobacteriaceae infections.*)

Causes

Although some strains of *E. coli* exist as part of the normal GI flora, infection usually results from certain nonindigenous strains. For example, noninvasive diarrhea results from two toxins produced by strains called enterotoxic or enteropathogenic *E. coli.* These toxins interact with intestinal juices and promote excessive loss of chloride and water. In the invasive form, *E. coli* directly invades the intestinal mucosa without producing enterotoxins, thereby causing local irritation, inflammation, and diarrhea. Normal strains can cause infection in immunocompromised patients.

Transmission can occur directly from an infected person or indirectly by ingestion of contaminated food or water or contact with contaminated utensils. Incubation takes 12 to 72 hours.

Incidence of *E. coli* infection is highest among travelers returning from other countries, particularly Mexico, Southeast Asia, and South America. *E. coli* infection also induces other diseases, especially in people whose resistance is low. A new strain, *E. coli* 0157:H7, is associated with undercooked hamburger.

Signs and symptoms

Effects of noninvasive diarrhea depend on the toxin causing the infection but may include the abrupt onset of watery diarrhea with cramping abdominal pain and, in severe illness, acidosis. Invasive infection produces chills, abdominal cramps, and diarrheic stools that may contain blood and pus.

Infantile diarrhea resulting from an *E. coli* infection is usually noninvasive; it begins with loose, watery stools that change from yellow to green and contain little mucus or blood. Vomiting, listlessness, irritability, and anorexia often precede diarrhea, which may progress to fever, severe dehydration, acidosis, and shock. Bloody diarrhea may occur with the *E. coli* 0157:H7 strain.

Diagnosis

Because certain strains of *E. coli* are normally present in the GI tract, culturing is of little value; diagnosis depends on clinical observation. Firm diagnosis requires sophisticated identification procedures, such as bioassays, that are expensive, time-consuming, and, consequently, not widely available. Diagnosis must rule out salmonellosis and shigellosis, other common infections that typically produce similar signs and symptoms.

Treatment

Appropriate treatment consists of isolation and correction of fluid and electrolyte imbalance; in an infant or immunocompromised patient, I.V. antibiotics based on the organism's drug sensitivity; and magnesium salicylate or tincture of opium for cramping and diarrhea.

Special considerations

• Keep accurate intake and output records. Measure stool volume and note presence of blood and pus. Replace fluids and electrolytes as needed, monitoring for decreased serum sodium and chloride levels and signs of gram-negative shock. Watch for signs of dehydration, such as poor skin turgor and dry mouth.
• For infants, provide isolation, give nothing by mouth, administer antibiotics, and maintain body warmth.
• To prevent spread of this infection, screen all hospital personnel and visitors for diarrhea, and prevent direct patient contact during epidemics. Report cases to local public health authorities.
• Use proper hand-washing technique. Teach personnel, patients, and their families to do the same.

• Use enteric precautions: private room, gown and gloves while handling feces, and hand washing before entering and after leaving the patient's room.
• Advise travelers to foreign countries to avoid unbottled water and uncooked vegetables.
• To prevent accumulation of these water-loving organisms, discard suction bottles, irrigating fluid, and open bottles of saline solution every 24 hours. Be sure to change I.V. tubing according to hospital policy and empty ventilator water reservoirs before refilling with sterile water. Remember to use suction catheters only once.

Pseudomonas infections

Nosocomial infections, superinfections of various parts of the body, and a rare disease called melioidosis are caused by *Pseudomonas,* a small, gram-negative bacillus. This bacillus is also associated with bacteremia, endocarditis, and osteo-myelitis in drug addicts. In local *Pseudomonas* infections, treatment is usually successful and complications rare. However, in immunocompromised patients – premature infants, elderly people, or those with debilitating diseases, burns, or wounds – septicemic *Pseudomonas* infections are serious and sometimes fatal. (See *Melioidosis,* page 64.)

Causes
The most common species of *Pseudomonas* is *P. aeruginosa.* Other species that typically cause disease in humans include *P. acidovorans, P. alcaligenes, P. cepacia, P. fluorescens, P. maltophilia, P. putida, P. putrefaciens, P. stutzeri,* and *P. testosteroni.* These organisms are frequently found in hospital liquids that have been allowed to stand for a long time, such as benzalkonium chloride, hexachlorophene soap, saline solution, penicillin, water in flower vases, and fluids in incubators, humidifiers, and inhalation therapy equipment.

In elderly patients, *Pseudomonas* organisms usually enter through the genitourinary tract; in infants, through the umbilical cord, skin, and GI tract.

Melioidosis

Wound penetration, inhalation, or ingestion of the gram-negative bacteria *Pseudomonas pseudomallei* causes melioidosis. Once confined to Southeast Asia, Central America, South America, Madagascar, and Guam, incidence in the United States is rising due to the recent influx of Southeast Asians.

Two forms

Melioidosis occurs in two forms: chronic melioidosis, causing osteomyelitis and lung abscesses; and acute melioidosis, which is rare, causing pneumonia, bacteremia, and prostration. Acute melioidosis is often fatal. However, most infections are chronic and asymptomatic, producing clinical symptoms only with accompanying malnutrition, major surgery, or severe burns.

Diagnosis and treatment

Diagnostic measures consist of isolation of *P. pseudomallei* in a culture of exudate, blood, or sputum; serologic tests (complement fixation, passive hemagglutination); and chest X-ray (findings resemble tuberculosis).

Treatment includes oral tetracycline, co-trimoxazole, abscess drainage in severe cases, and chloramphenicol until X-rays show resolution of primary abscesses.

The prognosis is good because most patients have mild infections and acquire permanent immunity; also, aggressive use of antibiotics and sulfonamides has improved the prognosis in acute melioidosis.

Signs and symptoms

The most common infections associated with *Pseudomonas* include skin infections (such as burns and pressure ulcers), urinary tract infections, infant epidemic diarrhea and other diarrheic illnesses, bronchitis, pneumonia, bronchiectasis, meningitis, corneal ulcers, mastoiditis, otitis externa, otitis media, endocarditis, and bacteremia.

Drainage in *Pseudomonas* infections has a distinct, sickly sweet odor and contains a greenish blue pus that forms a crust on wounds. Other symptoms depend on the site of infection. For example, when it invades the lungs, *Pseudomonas* causes pneumonia with fever, chills, and a productive cough.

Diagnosis

Accurate diagnosis of *Pseudomonas* infection requires isolation of the organism in blood, spinal fluid, urine, exudate, or sputum culture.

Treatment

In the debilitated or otherwise vulnerable patient with clinical evidence of *Pseudomonas* infection, treatment should begin immediately, without waiting for results of laboratory tests. Antibiotic treatment includes aminoglycosides, such as gentamicin or tobramycin, combined with a *Pseudomonas*-sensitive penicillin, such as carbenicillin disodium or ticarcillin. An alternative combination is amikacin and a similar penicillin or ciprofloxacin. Such combination therapy is necessary because *Pseudomonas* quickly becomes resistant to carbenicillin alone. However, in urinary tract infections, carbenicillin indanyl sodium or ciprofloxacin can be used alone if the organism is susceptible and the infection doesn't have systemic effects; both drugs are excreted in urine and build up high urine levels that prevent resistance.

Local *Pseudomonas* infections or septicemia secondary to wound infection require 1% acetic acid irrigations, topical applications of colistimethate sodium and polymyxin B, and debridement or drainage of the infected wound.

Special considerations

• Observe and record the character of wound exudate and sputum.
• Before administering antibiotics, ask the patient about a history of allergies, especially to penicillin. If combinations of carbenicillin or ticarcillin and an aminoglycoside are ordered, schedule the doses 1 hour apart (carbenicillin and ticarcillin may decrease the antibiotic effect of the aminoglycoside). *Don't* give both antibiotics through the same administration set.
• Monitor the patient's renal function (urine output, blood urea nitrogen, specific gravity, urinalysis, creatinine) during treatment with aminoglycosides.
• Protect immunocompromised patients from exposure to this infection. Attention to hand washing and aseptic techniques prevents further spread.
• To prevent *Pseudomonas* infection, maintain proper endotracheal or tracheostomy suctioning technique: use strict sterile technique when caring for I.V. lines, catheters, and other tubes; dispose of suction bottle contents properly; and label and date solution bottles, and change them frequently according to hospital policy.

Vibrio parahaemolyticus food poisoning

Infection by *V. parahaemolyticus* is a common cause of gastroenteritis in Japan; outbreaks also occur on American cruise ships and in the eastern and southeastern coastal areas of the United States, especially during the summer.

V. parahaemolyticus, which thrives in a salty environment, is transmitted by ingesting uncooked or undercooked, contaminated shellfish, particularly crabs and shrimp.

Signs and symptoms
After an incubation period of 2 to 48 hours, *V. parahaemolyticus* causes watery diarrhea, moderately severe cramps, nausea, vomiting, headache, weakness, chills, and fever. Food poisoning is usually self-limiting and subsides spontaneously within 2 days.

Occasionally, however, it's more severe, and may even be fatal in debilitated or elderly people.

Diagnosis
A positive diagnosis requires bacteriologic examination of vomitus, blood, stool smears, or fecal specimens collected by rectal swab. Diagnosis must rule out not only other causes of food poisoning but also other acute GI disorders.

Supportive treatment
Appropriate treatment consists primarily of bed rest and oral fluid replacement. I.V. replacement therapy is seldom necessary, but oral tetracycline may be prescribed. Thorough cooking of seafood prevents this infection.

Cholera

Also called Asiatic cholera or epidemic cholera, cholera is an acute enterotoxin-mediated GI infection caused by the gram-negative rod *Vibrio cholerae.* It produces profuse diarrhea, vomiting, massive fluid and electrolyte losses, and possibly hypovolemic shock, metabolic acidosis, and death. A similar bacterium, *V. parahaemolyticus,* causes food poisoning. (See Vibrio parahaemolyticus *food poisoning.*)

Even with prompt diagnosis and treatment, cholera is fatal in up to 2% of children; in adults, it is fatal in fewer than 1%. However, untreated cholera may be fatal in as many as 50% of patients. Cholera infection confers only transient immunity.

Causes

Humans are the only hosts and victims of *V. cholerae*, a motile, aerobic rod. It's transmitted through food and water contaminated with fecal material from carriers or persons with active infections. Cholera is most common in Africa, southern and Southeast Asia, and the Middle East, although outbreaks have occurred in Japan, Australia, and Europe. A new epidemic is now occurring in western South America and parts of Central America.

Cholera occurs during the warmer months and is most prevalent among lower socioeconomic groups. In India, it's common among children ages 1 to 5, but in other endemic areas, it's equally distributed among all age-groups. Deficiency or absence of hydrochloric acid in gastric juices may increase susceptibility to cholera.

Signs and symptoms

After an incubation period ranging from several hours to 5 days, cholera produces acute, painless, profuse, watery diarrhea and effortless vomiting (without preceding nausea). As the number of stools increases, the stools contain white flecks of mucus ("rice-water stools"). Because of massive fluid and electrolyte losses from diarrhea and vomiting (fluid loss in adults may reach 1 liter/hour), cholera causes intense thirst, weakness, loss of skin turgor, wrinkled skin, sunken eyes, pinched facial expression, muscle cramps (especially in the extremities), cyanosis, oliguria, tachycardia, tachypnea, thready or absent peripheral pulses, falling blood pressure, fever, and inaudible, hypoactive bowel sounds.

Patients usually remain oriented but apathetic, although small children may become stuporous or develop seizures. If complications don't occur, the symptoms subside and the patient recovers within a week. But if treatment is delayed or inadequate, cholera may lead to metabolic acidosis, uremia, and possibly coma and death. About 3% of patients who recover continue to carry *V. cholerae* in the gallbladder; however, most patients are free of the infection after about 2 weeks.

Diagnosis

In endemic areas or during epidemics, typical clinical features strongly suggest cholera. A culture of *V. cholerae* from feces or vomitus indicates cholera, but definitive diagnosis requires agglutination and other clear reactions to group and type-specific antisera. A dark-field microscopic examination of fresh feces showing rapidly moving bacilli (like shooting stars) allows for a quick, tentative diagnosis.

C. Davis

Immunofluorescence also allows a rapid diagnosis. The diagnosis must rule out *Escherichia coli* infection, salmonellosis, and shigellosis.

Treatment

Improved sanitation and the administration of cholera vaccine to travelers in endemic areas can control this disease. Unfortunately, the vaccine now available confers only 60% to 80% immunity and is effective for only 3 to 6 months. Consequently, vaccination is impractical for residents of endemic areas.

Treatment requires dehydration by rapid I.V. infusion of large amounts (50 to 100 ml/minute) of isotonic saline solution, alternating with isotonic sodium bicarbonate or sodium lactate. Potassium replacement may be added to the I.V. solution.

When I.V. infusions have corrected hypovolemia, fluid infusion decreases to quantities sufficient to maintain normal pulse and skin turgor or to replace liquid loss through diarrhea. An oral glucose electrolyte solution can substitute for I.V. infusions. In mild cholera, oral fluid replacement is adequate. If symptoms persist despite fluid and electrolyte replacement, treatment includes tetracycline.

Special considerations

• Follow enteric precautions, give supportive care, and closely observe the patient during the acute phase of the disease.
• Wear a gown and gloves when handling feces-contaminated articles or when a danger of contaminating clothing exists, and wash your hands after leaving the patient's room.
• Monitor output (including stool volume) and I.V. infusion accurately. To detect overhydration, carefully observe neck veins and auscultate the lungs. (Fluid loss in cholera is massive, and improper replacement may cause potentially fatal renal insufficiency.)
• Protect the patient's family by administering oral tetracycline if necessary.
• Advise anyone traveling to an endemic area to boil all drinking water and avoid uncooked vegetables and unpeeled fruits. If the doctor orders a cholera vaccine, tell the patient that he'll need a booster inoculation 3 to 6 months later for continuing protection.

Septic shock

Second only to cardiogenic shock as the leading cause of shock-related death, septic shock (usually a result of bacterial infection) causes inadequate tissue perfusion, abnormalities of oxygen supply and demand, metabolic changes, and circulatory collapse. It occurs most often among hospitalized patients. About 25% of patients who develop gram-negative bacteremia go into shock. Unless vigorous treatment begins promptly, preferably before symptoms fully develop, septic shock rapidly progresses to death (often within a few hours) in up to 80% of these patients.

Causes

In two-thirds of patients, septic shock results from infection with gram-negative bacteria: *Escherichia coli, Klebsiella, Enterobacter, Proteus, Pseudomonas,* and *Bacteroides;* in a few, from gram-positive bacteria: *Streptococcus pneumoniae, S. pyogenes,* and *Actinomyces.* Infections with viruses, rickettsiae, chlamydiae, and protozoa may be complicated by shock.

These organisms produce septicemia in people whose resistance is already compromised by an existing condition; infection also results from transplantation of bacteria from other areas of the body through surgery, I.V. therapy, and catheters. Septic shock often occurs in patients hospitalized for primary infection of the genitourinary, biliary, GI, and gynecologic tracts. Other predisposing factors include immunodeficiency, advanced age, trauma, burns, diabetes mellitus, cirrhosis, and disseminated cancer.

Signs and symptoms

The symptoms of septic shock vary according to the stage of the shock, the organism causing it, and the patient's immune response and age:
• Early stage: oliguria, sudden fever (over 101° F [38.3° C]), and chills; tachypnea, tachycardia, full bounding pulse, hyperglycemia, nausea, vomiting, diarrhea, and prostration
• Late stage: restlessness, apprehension, irritability, thirst from decreased cerebral tissue perfusion, hypoglycemia, hypothermia, and anuria. Hypotension, altered level of con-

sciousness, and hyperventilation may be the *only* signs among infants and the elderly.

Complications of septic shock include disseminated intravascular coagulation (DIC), renal failure, heart failure, GI ulcers, and hepatic dysfunction.

Diagnosis

One or more typical symptoms (fever, confusion, nausea, vomiting, hyperventilation) in a patient suspected of having an infection suggests septic shock and necessitates immediate treatment.

In early stages, arterial blood gas (ABG) analysis indicates respiratory alkalosis (low $PaCO_2$, low or normal bicarbonate, high pH); as shock progresses, metabolic acidosis develops with hypoxemia indicated by decreasing $PaCO_2$ (may increase as respiratory failure ensues), PaO_2, HCO_3^-, and pH. The following tests support the diagnosis and determine the treatment:
• blood cultures to isolate the organism
• decreased platelet count and leukocytosis (15,000 to 30,000/ mm^3)
• increased blood urea nitrogen and creatinine levels, and decreased creatinine clearance
• abnormal prothrombin time and partial thromboplastin time
• simultaneous measurement of urine and plasma osmolalities for renal failure (urine osmolality below 400 mOsm, with a ratio of urine to plasma below 1.5)
• decreased central venous pressure (CVP), pulmonary artery and wedge pressures, and cardiac output (although in early septic shock, cardiac output increases); low systemic vascular resistance
• electrocardiogram – ST-segment depression, inverted T waves, and arrhythmia resembling myocardial infarction.

Treatment

The first goal of treatment is to monitor and reverse shock through volume expansion with I.V. fluids and insertion of a pulmonary artery catheter to check pulmonary arterial wedge pressure (PAWP). Administration of whole blood or plasma can then raise the PAWP to a high-normal to slightly elevated level of 14 to 18 mm Hg. A respirator may be necessary for proper ventilation to overcome hypoxia. Urinary catheterization allows accurate measurement of hourly urine output.

Treatment also requires immediate administration of I.V. antibiotics to control the infection. Depending on the organism, the antibiotic combination usually includes an aminoglycoside (such as amikacin, gentamicin, or tobramycin) for gram-negative bacteria, combined with a penicillin (such as carbenicillin, ticarcillin, or piperacillin).

Sometimes treatment includes a cephalosporin (such as cefazolin, vancomycin, or nafcillin) for suspected staphylococcal infection instead of carbenicillin or ticarcillin. Therapy may include chloramphenicol for nonsporulating anaerobes *(Bacteroides)*, although it may cause bone marrow depression, and clindamycin, which may produce pseudomembranous enterocolitis. Appropriate antibiotics for other causes of septic shock depend on the suspected organism. Other measures to combat infections include surgery to drain and excise abscesses, and debridement.

If shock persists after fluid infusion, treatment with vasopressors, such as dopamine, maintains adequate blood perfusion in the brain, liver, digestive tract, kidneys, and skin. Other treatment includes I.V. bicarbonate to correct acidosis. A new gram-negative endotoxin vaccine has been used with some success. Other experimental treatments include corticosteroids, opiate antagonists, prostaglandin inhibitors, and calcium channel blockers, which are used to block the rapid inflammatory process.

Special considerations

• Determine which of your patients are at high risk for developing septic shock.
• Know the signs of impending septic shock, but don't rely solely on technical aids to judge the patient's status. Consider any change in mental status and urinary output as significant as a change in CVP.
• Carefully maintain the pulmonary artery catheter. Remember to check ABG levels for adequate oxygenation or gas exchange.
• Record intake and output and daily weight. Maintain urine output (0.5 to 1 ml/kg/hour) and adequate systolic pressure. Avoid fluid overload.
• Monitor serum antibiotic levels and administer drugs.
• Watch the patient closely for signs of DIC (abnormal bleeding); renal failure (oliguria, increased specific gravity); heart failure (dyspnea, edema, tachycardia, distended neck veins);

GI ulcers (hematemesis, melena); and hepatic abnormality (jaundice, hypoprothrombinemia, and hypoalbuminemia).

Haemophilus influenzae infection

A small, gram-negative, pleomorphic aerobic bacillus, *Haemophilus influenzae* appears predominantly coccobacillary in exudates. It causes diseases in many organ systems but most frequently attacks the respiratory system. It's a common cause of epiglottitis, laryngotracheobronchitis, pneumonia, bronchiolitis, otitis media, and meningitis. Less often, it causes bacterial endocarditis, conjunctivitis, facial cellulitis, septic arthritis, and osteomyelitis. *H. influenzae* pneumonia is an increasingly common nosocomial infection. It infects about half of all children before age 1 and virtually all children by age 3, although a new vaccine given at ages 2, 4, and 6 months has reduced this number.

Signs and symptoms

H. influenzae provokes a characteristic tissue response — acute suppurative inflammation. When *H. influenzae* infects the larynx, the trachea, and the bronchial tree, it leads to mucosal edema and thick exudate; when it invades the lungs, it leads to bronchopneumonia. In the pharynx, *H. influenzae* usually produces no remarkable changes, except when it causes epiglottitis, which generally affects both the laryngeal and the pharyngeal surfaces. The pharyngeal mucosa may be reddened, rarely with soft yellow exudate. More likely, however, it appears normal or shows only slight diffuse redness, even while severe pain makes swallowing difficult or impossible. These infections typically cause high fever and generalized malaise.

Diagnosis

Isolation of the organism confirms *H. influenzae* infection, usually with a blood culture. Other laboratory findings include:
• polymorphonuclear leukocytosis (15,000 to 30,000/mm^3)
• leukopenia (2,000 to 3,000/mm^3) in young children with severe infection

• *H. influenzae* bacteremia, found frequently in patients with meningitis.

Treatment

H. influenzae infections usually respond to a 2-week course of ampicillin (resistant strains are becoming more common), cephalosporins, or chloramphenicol.

Special considerations

• Maintain adequate respiratory function through proper positioning, humidification (such as a croup tent) in children, and suctioning as needed. Monitor rate and type of respirations. Watch for signs of cyanosis and dyspnea, because they necessitate intubation or a tracheotomy. Monitor level of consciousness (LOC). Decreased LOC may indicate hypoxemia. For home treatment, suggest using a room humidifier or breathing moist air from a shower or bath as necessary.
• Check the patient's history for drug allergies before administering antibiotics. Monitor complete blood count for signs of bone marrow depression when therapy includes ampicillin or chloramphenicol.
• Monitor intake (including I.V. infusions) and output. Watch for signs of dehydration, such as decreased skin turgor, parched lips, concentrated urine, decreased urine output, and increased pulse.
• Organize your physical care measures beforehand, and do them quickly so as not to disrupt the patient's rest.
• Take preventive measures, such as giving the *H. influenzae* vaccine to children age 2 (or younger) to 6, maintaining respiratory isolation, using proper hand-washing technique, properly disposing of respiratory secretions, placing soiled tissues in a plastic bag, and decontaminating all equipment.

Pertussis

A highly contagious respiratory infection, pertussis (whooping cough) is usually caused by the nonmotile, gram-negative coccobacillus *Bordetella pertussis,* and, occasionally, by the related similar bacteria *B. parapertussis* and *B. bronchiseptica.* Characteristically, pertussis produces an irritating cough that becomes paroxysmal and often ends in a high-pitched, inspiratory whoop.

Since the 1940s, immunization and aggressive diagnosis and treatment have significantly reduced mortality from pertussis in North America. Mortality in children under age 1 is usually a result of pneumonia and other complications. Pertussis is also dangerous in the elderly but tends to be less severe in older children and adults.

Causes

Pertussis is usually transmitted by the direct inhalation of contaminated droplets from a patient in the acute stage; it may also be spread indirectly through soiled linen and other articles contaminated by respiratory secretions.

Pertussis is endemic throughout the world and usually occurs in early spring and late winter. About half the time, it strikes unimmunized children under age 2, probably because women of childbearing age don't usually have high serum levels of *B. pertussis* antibodies to transmit to their offspring.

Signs and symptoms

After an incubation period of about 7 to 10 days, *B. pertussis* enters the tracheobronchial mucosa, where it produces progressively tenacious mucus. Pertussis follows a classic 6-week course that includes three stages, each of which lasts about 2 weeks.

First, the catarrhal stage characteristically produces an irritating, hacking, nocturnal cough; anorexia; sneezing; listlessness; infected conjunctivae; and, occasionally, a low-grade fever. This stage is highly communicable.

After a period of 7 to 14 days, the paroxysmal stage produces spasmodic and recurrent coughing that may expel tenacious mucus. Each cough characteristically ends in a loud, crowing inspiratory whoop, and choking on mucus causes vomiting. (Very young infants, however, might not develop the typical whoop.) Paroxysmal coughing may induce complications, such as increased venous pressure, nosebleed, periorbital edema, conjunctival hemorrhage, hemorrhage of the anterior chamber of the eye, detached retina (and blindness), rectal prolapse, inguinal or umbilical hernia, convulsions, atelectasis, and pneumonitis. In infants, choking spells may cause apnea, anoxia, and disturbed acid-base balance. During this stage, patients are highly vulnerable to fatal secondary bacterial or viral infections. Suspect such secondary infection (usually otitis media or pneumonia) in any pertussis patient with a fever during this stage, because pertussis itself seldom causes fever.

During the convalescent stage, paroxysmal coughing and vomiting gradually subside. However, for months afterward, even a mild upper respiratory infection may trigger paroxysmal coughing.

Diagnosis

Classic clinical findings, especially during the paroxysmal stage, suggest this diagnosis; laboratory studies confirm it. Nasopharyngeal swabs and sputum cultures show *B. pertussis* only in the early stages of this disease; fluorescent antibody screening of nasopharyngeal smears provides quicker results than cultures but is less reliable. In addition, white blood cell (WBC) count is usually increased, especially in children older than 6 months and early in the paroxysmal stage. Sometimes, the WBC count may reach 175,000 to 200,000/mm^3, with 60% to 90% lymphocytes.

Treatment

Vigorous supportive therapy requires hospitalization of infants (often in the intensive care unit), and fluid and electrolyte replacement. Other treatment includes adequate nutrition; codeine and mild sedation to decrease coughing; oxygen therapy (in apnea); and antibiotics, such as erythromycin and, possibly, ampicillin, to shorten the period of communicability and prevent secondary infections.

Because infants are particularly susceptible to pertussis, immunization — usually with diphtheria and tetanus toxoids — takes place at 2, 4, and 6 months. Booster inoculations follow at 18 months and at 4 to 6 years. The risk of pertussis exceeds the risk of vaccine complications such as neurologic damage. However, if vaccination causes seizures or unusual and persistent crying, this may signal a severe neurologic reaction; additional doses may not be given. The vaccine is contraindicated in children over age 6, because it can cause a high fever.

Special considerations

• Pertussis calls for aggressive supportive care and respiratory isolation (masks only) for 5 to 7 days after initiation of antibiotic therapy.
• Monitor acid-base, fluid, and electrolyte balance.

• Carefully suction secretions and monitor oxygen therapy. Remember: Suctioning removes oxygen as well as secretions.
• Create a quiet environment to decrease coughing stimulation. Provide small, frequent meals, and treat constipation or nausea caused by codeine.
• Offer emotional support to parents of children with pertussis.
• To decrease exposure to organisms, make sure that soiled linen are changed, suction bottle emptied, and trash bag changed at least once every 8 hours.

Plague

An acute infection, plague (black death) is caused by the gram-negative, nonmotile, nonsporulating bacillus *Yersinia pestis* (formerly called *Pasteurella pestis*).

Plague occurs in several forms. Bubonic plague, the most common, causes the characteristic swollen, and sometimes suppurating, lymph glands (buboes) that give this infection its name. Other forms include septicemic plague, a severe, rapid systemic form, and pneumonic plague, which can be primary or secondary to the other two forms. Primary pneumonic plague is an acutely fulminant, highly contagious form that causes acute prostration, respiratory distress, and death—often within 2 to 3 days after onset.

Without treatment, mortality is about 60% in bubonic plague and approaches 100% in both septicemic and pneumonic plagues. With treatment, reported mortality is approximately 18% and is related to the delay between onset and treatment and to the patient's age and physical condition.

Causes

Plague is usually transmitted to a human through the bite of a flea from an infected rodent host, such as a rat, squirrel, prairie dog, or hare. Occasionally, transmission occurs when infected animals or their tissues are handled.

Bubonic plague is notorious for the historic pandemics in Europe and Asia during the Middle Ages, which in some areas killed up to two-thirds of the population. This form is rarely transmitted from person to person. However, the untreated bubonic form may progress to a secondary pneumonic form, which is transmitted by contaminated respiratory droplets (coughing) and is highly contagious. The 1994 outbreak in India underscored this pattern of contagion.

In the United States, the primary pneumonic form usually occurs after inhalation of *Y. pestis* in a laboratory. Sylvatic (wild rodent) plague remains endemic to South America, the Near East, central and Southeast Asia, north central and southern Africa, Mexico, and the western United States and Canada. In the United States, its incidence has been rising, a possible reflection of different bacterial strains or environmental changes that favor rodent growth in certain areas. Plague tends to occur between May and September; between October and February it usually occurs in hunters who skin wild animals. One attack confers permanent immunity.

Signs and symptoms

The incubation period, early symptoms, severity at onset, and clinical course vary in the three forms of plague. In bubonic plague, the incubation period is 2 to 6 days. The milder form begins with malaise, fever, and pain or tenderness in regional lymph nodes, possibly associated with swelling. Lymph node damage (usually axillary or inguinal) eventually produces painful, inflamed, and possibly suppurative buboes. The classic sign of plague is an excruciatingly painful bubo. Hemorrhagic areas may become necrotic; in the skin, such areas appear dark—hence the name "black death." This infection can progress extremely rapidly: A seemingly mildly ill person with symptoms limited to fever and adenitis may become moribund within hours. Plague may also begin dramatically, with a sudden high temperature of 103° to 106° F (39.4° to 41.1°C), chills, myalgia, headache, prostration, restlessness, disorientation, delirium, toxemia, and staggering gait. Occasionally, it causes abdominal pain, nausea, vomiting, and constipation, followed by diarrhea (frequently bloody), skin mottling, petechiae, and circulatory collapse.

In primary pneumonic plague, the incubation period is 2 to 3 days, followed by a typically acute onset, with high fever, chills, severe headache, tachycardia, tachypnea, dyspnea, and a productive cough (first, mucoid sputum; later, frothy pink or red).

Secondary pneumonic plague, the pulmonary extension of the bubonic form, complicates about 5% of untreated plague. A cough producing bloody sputum signals this complication. Primary and secondary pneumonic plagues rapidly cause severe prostration, respiratory distress, and possibly death.

Septicemic plague usually develops without overt lymph node enlargement. In this form, the patient shows toxicity, hyperpyrexia, convulsions, prostration, shock, and disseminated intravascular coagulation (DIC). Septicemic plague causes widespread nonspecific tissue damage — such as peritoneal or pleural effusion, pericarditis, and meningitis — and is rapidly fatal unless promptly and correctly treated.

Diagnosis

Because plague is rare in North America, it's often overlooked until after the patient dies or multiple cases develop. Characteristic buboes and a history of exposure to rodents strongly suggest bubonic plague.

Stained smears and cultures of Y. pestis obtained from a needle aspirate of a small amount of fluid from skin lesions confirm this diagnosis.

Postmortem examination of a guinea pig inoculated with a sample of blood or purulent drainage allows isolation of the organism. Other laboratory studies include white blood cell count increased to over 20,000/mm^3 with increased polymorphonuclear leukocytes, and hemagglutination reaction (antibody titer) studies. Diagnosis should rule out tularemia, typhus, and typhoid.

In pneumonic plague, diagnosis requires a chest X-ray to show fulminating pneumonia, and stained smear and culture of sputum to identify Y. pestis. Other bacterial pneumonias and psittacosis must be ruled out. Stained smear and blood culture containing Y. pestis are diagnostic in septicemic plague. However, because cultures of Y. pestis grow slowly, in suspected plague (especially pneumonic and septicemic plagues), treatment should begin without waiting for laboratory confirmation. For a presumptive diagnosis of plague, a fluorescent antibody test may be ordered.

Treatment

Antimicrobial treatment of suspected plague must begin immediately after blood specimens have been taken for culture and shouldn't be delayed for laboratory confirmation. Generally, treatment consists of large doses of streptomycin, the drug proven most effective against *Y. pestis*. Other effective drugs include tetracycline, chloramphenicol, kanamycin, and possibly co-trimoxazole. Penicillins are ineffective against plague.

In both septicemic and pneumonic plagues, lifesaving antimicrobial treatment must begin within 18 hours of onset. Supportive management aims to control fever, shock, and convulsions and to maintain fluid balance.

After antimicrobial therapy has begun, glucocorticoids can combat life-threatening toxemia and shock; diazepam relieves restlessness; and if the patient develops DIC, treatment may include heparin.

Special considerations

• Patients with plague require strict isolation, which may be discontinued 48 hours after antimicrobial therapy begins unless respiratory symptoms develop.
• Use an approved insecticide to rid patient and clothing of fleas. Carefully dispose of soiled dressings and linens, feces, and sputum. If patient has pneumonic plague, wear a gown, mask, and gloves. Handle all exudates, purulent discharges, and laboratory specimens with rubber gloves. For more information, consult your infection control officer.
• Give drugs and treat complications.
• Treat buboes with hot, moist compresses. Never excise or drain them because this may spread the infection.
• When septicemic plague causes peripheral tissue necrosis, prevent further injury to necrotic tissue. Avoid using restraints or arm boards, and pad the side rails.
• Obtain a history of patient contacts for a quarantine of 6 days of observation. Administer prophylactic tetracycline as needed.
• Report suspected cases to local public health department officials so they can identify the source of infection.
• To help prevent plague, discourage contact with wild animals (especially those that are sick or dead), and support

programs aimed at reducing insect and rodent populations. • Recommend immunization with plague vaccine to travelers to or residents of endemic areas, even though the effect of immunization is transient.

Brucellosis

An acute febrile illness, brucellosis (also called undulant fever, Malta fever, febris melitensis, and Mediterranean fever) is transmitted to humans from animals, and is caused by the non-motile, non-spore-forming, gram-negative coccobacilli *Brucella* bacteria, notably *B. suis* (found in swine), *B. melitensis* (in goats), *B. abortus* (in cattle), and *B. canis* (in dogs). Brucellosis causes fever, profuse sweating, anxiety, achiness, and bone, spleen, liver, kidney, or brain abscesses. The prognosis is good: With treatment, brucellosis is rarely fatal, although complications may cause permanent disability.

Causes

Brucellosis is transmitted through the consumption of unpasteurized dairy products or uncooked or undercooked contaminated meat, and through contact with infected animals, their secretions, or excretions. It's most common among farmers, stock handlers, butchers, and veterinarians. Because of these occupational risks, brucellosis infects men six times more often than it does women, especially those between ages 20 and 50; it's less common in children. Since hydrochloric acid in gastric juices kills *Brucella* bacteria, persons with achlorhydria are particularly susceptible to this disease.

Although brucellosis occurs throughout the world, it's most prevalent in the Middle East, Africa, Russia, India, South America, and Europe; it's rarely found in the United States. The incubation period is usually from 5 to 35 days, but in some cases it can last for months.

Signs and symptoms

Onset of brucellosis is usually insidious, but the disease course falls into two distinct phases. Characteristically, the acute phase causes fever, chills, profuse sweating, fatigue, headache, backache, enlarged lymph nodes, hepatospleno-megaly, weight loss, and abscess and granuloma formation in subcutaneous tissues, lymph nodes, the liver, and the spleen. Despite this disease's common name, undulant fever, few patients have a truly undulant (intermittent) fever; in fact, fever is often insignificant.

The chronic phase produces recurrent depression, sleep disturbances, fatigue, headache, sweating, and sexual impotence; hepatosplenomegaly and enlarged lymph nodes persist. In addition, abscesses may form in the testes, ovaries, kidneys, and brain (meningitis and encephalitis). About 10% to 15% of patients with brain abscesses develop hearing and visual disorders, hemiplegia, and ataxia. Other complications include osteomyelitis, orchitis and, rarely, subacute infective endocarditis, which is difficult to treat.

Diagnosis

In patients with characteristic clinical features, a history of exposure to animals suggests brucellosis. Multiple agglutinin tests help to confirm the diagnosis.
• Approximately 90% of patients with brucellosis have agglutinin titers of 1:160 or more within 3 weeks of developing this disease. However, elevated agglutinin titers also follow vaccination against tularemia, *Yersinia* infection, or cholera; skin tests; or relapse. Agglutinin testing can also monitor the effectiveness of treatment.
• Multiple (three to six) cultures of blood and bone marrow and biopsies of infected tissue (for example, the spleen) provide a definite diagnosis. Culturing is best done during the acute phase.
• Blood studies indicate an increased erythrocyte sedimentation rate and normal or reduced white blood count.

Diagnosis must rule out infectious diseases that produce similar symptoms, such as typhoid and malaria.

Treatment

Appropriate treatment consists of bed rest during the febrile phase; a 3-week course of oral tetracycline with a 2-week course of streptomycin I.M.; and, in severe cases, corticosteroids I.V. for 3 days, followed by oral corticosteroids. Secretion precautions are required until lesions stop draining.

Special
considerations

• In suspected brucellosis, take a full history. Ask the patient about his occupation and if he has recently traveled abroad or eaten unprocessed food such as goat's milk.
• During the acute phase, monitor and record the patient's temperature every 4 hours. Be sure to use the same route (oral or rectal) every time. Ask the dietary department to provide between-meal milk shakes and other supplemental foods to counter weight loss. Watch for heart murmurs, muscle weakness, vision loss, and joint inflammation – all may point to complications.
• During the chronic phase, watch for depression and disturbed sleep patterns. Administer sedatives and plan your care to allow adequate rest.
• Keep suppurative granulomas and abscesses dry. Double-bag and properly dispose of all secretions and soiled dressings. Reassure the patient that this infection *is* curable.
• Before discharge, stress the importance of continuing medication for the prescribed duration.
• To prevent recurrence, advise patients to cook meat thoroughly and avoid using unpasteurized milk. Warn meat packers and other persons at risk for occupational exposure to wear rubber gloves and goggles.

SPIROCHETES AND MYCOBACTERIA

Diseases caused by spirochetes and mycobacteria may advance from mild to incapacitating and life-threatening. Most progress in stages and all affect skin integrity to some extent.

Lyme disease

A multisystemic disorder, Lyme disease is caused by the spirochete *Borrelia burgdorferi,* which is carried by the minute tick *Ixodes dammini* or another tick in the Ixodidae family. It often begins in the summer with the classic skin lesion called erythema chronicum migrans (ECM). Weeks or months later, cardiac or neurologic abnormalities may develop, possibly followed by arthritis.

Initially, Lyme disease was identified in a group of children in Lyme, Connecticut. Now Lyme disease is known to occur primarily in three parts of the United States: in the Northeast from Massachusetts to Maryland; in the Midwest, in Wisconsin and Minnesota; and in the West, in California and Oregon. Although it's endemic to these areas, cases have been reported in 43 states and 20 other countries, including Germany, Switzerland, France, and Australia.

Causes

Lyme disease occurs when a tick injects spirochete-laden saliva into the bloodstream or deposits fecal matter on the skin. After incubating for 3 to 32 days, the spirochetes migrate out to the skin, causing ECM. Then they disseminate to other skin sites or organs by the bloodstream or lymphatic system. The spirochetes' life cycle isn't completely clear: They may survive for years in the joints or they may trigger an inflammatory response in the host and then die.

Signs and symptoms

Typically, Lyme disease has three stages. ECM heralds stage one with a red macule or papule, often at the site of a tick bite. This lesion often feels hot and itchy and may grow to over 20″ (50 cm) in diameter. Within a few days, more lesions may erupt and a migratory, ringlike rash, conjunctivitis, or diffuse urticaria occurs. In 3 to 4 weeks, lesions are replaced by small red blotches, which persist for several more weeks. Malaise and fatigue are constant, but other findings are intermittent: headache, fever, chills, achiness, and regional lymphadenopathy. Less common effects are meningeal irritation, mild encephalopathy, migrating musculoskeletal pain, and hepatitis. A persistent sore throat and dry cough may appear several days before ECM.

Weeks to months later, the second stage begins with neurologic abnormalities—fluctuating meningoencephalitis with peripheral and cranial neuropathy—that usually resolve after days or months. Facial palsy is especially noticeable. Cardiac abnormalities, such as a brief, fluctuating atrioventricular heart block, may also develop.

Stage three begins weeks or years later and is characterized by arthritis. Migrating musculoskeletal pain leads to frank arthritis with marked swelling, especially in the large joints. Recurrent attacks may precede chronic arthritis with severe cartilage and bone erosion.

Diagnosis

Because isolation of *B. burgdorferi* is unusual in humans and because indirect immunofluorescent antibody tests are marginally sensitive, diagnosis often rests on the characteristic ECM lesion and related clinical findings, especially in endemic areas. Mild anemia and an elevated erythrocyte sedimentation rate, leukocyte count, and serum immunoglobulin and aspartate aminotransferase levels support the diagnosis.

Treatment

A 10- to 20-day course of oral tetracycline is the treatment of choice for adults. Penicillin and erythromycin are alternatives. Oral penicillin is usually prescribed for children. When given in the early stages, these drugs can minimize later complications. When given during the late stages, high-dose penicillin I.V. may be a successful treatment.

Special considerations

• Take a detailed patient history, asking about travel to endemic areas and exposure to ticks.
• Check for drug allergies and administer antibiotics carefully.
• For a patient with arthritis, help with range-of-motion and strengthening exercises, but avoid overexertion.
• Assess the patient's neurologic function and level of consciousness frequently. Watch for signs of increased intracranial pressure and cranial nerve involvement, such as ptosis, strabismus, and diplopia. Also check for cardiac abnormalities, such as arrhythmias and heart block.

Relapsing fever

An acute infectious disease caused by spirochetes of the genus *Borrelia,* relapsing fever is transmitted to humans by lice or ticks and is characterized by relapses and remissions. (Other names for relapsing fever include tick, recurrent, or famine fever.)

Rodents and other wild animals serve as the primary reservoirs for the *Borrelia* spirochetes. Humans can become secondary reservoirs but cannot transmit this infection by ordinary contagion; however, congenital infection and transmission by contaminated blood are possible.

Untreated louse-borne relapsing fever normally has a mortality of more than 10%. However, during an epidemic, mortality may rise to as high as 50%. The victims are usually indigent people who are already suffering from other infections and malnutrition. With treatment, however, the prognosis for both louse- and tick-borne relapsing fevers is excellent.

Causes

The body louse *(Pediculus humanis* var. *corporis)* carries louse-borne relapsing fever, which often erupts epidemically during wars, famines, and mass migrations. Cold weather and crowded living conditions also favor the spread of body lice.

Inoculation takes place when the victim crushes the louse, causing its infected blood or body fluid to soak into the victim's bitten or abraded skin or mucous membranes.

Louse-borne relapsing fever occurs most often in northern and central Africa, Europe, Asia, and South America. No cases of louse-borne relapsing fever have been reported in the United States since 1900.

Tick-borne relapsing fever, however, is found in the United States and is caused by three species of *Borrelia* most closely identified with tick carriers: *B. hermsii* with *Ornithodoros hermsi, B. turicatae* with *O. turicata,* and *B. parkeri* with *O. parkeri.* This disease is most prevalent in Texas and in other western states, usually during the summer, when ticks and their hosts (chipmunks, goats, prairie dogs) are most active. However, cold-weather outbreaks sometimes afflict persons, such as campers, who sleep in tick-infested cabins.

Because tick bites are virtually painless, and *Ornithodoros* ticks frequently feed at night but do not imbed themselves in the victim's skin, many people are bitten unknowingly.

Signs and symptoms

The incubation period for relapsing fever is 5 to 15 days (the average is 7 days). Clinically, tick- and louse-borne diseases are similar. Both begin suddenly, with a temperature approaching 105° F (40.5° C), prostration, headache, severe myalgia, arthralgia, diarrhea, vomiting, coughing, and eye or chest pains. Splenomegaly is common; hepatomegaly and lymphadenopathy are possible. During febrile periods, the victim's pulse rate and respiration rate rise, and a transient, macular rash may develop over his torso.

The first attack usually lasts from 3 to 6 days; then the patient experiences a quick drop in temperature, which is accompanied by profuse sweating. About 5 to 10 days later, a second febrile, symptomatic period begins. In louse-borne infection, additional relapses are unusual; but in tick-borne cases, a second or third relapse is common. As the afebrile intervals become longer, relapses become shorter and milder because of antibody accumulation. Relapses may be due to antigenic changes in the *Borrelia* organism.

Complications from relapsing fever include nephritis, bronchitis, pneumonia, endocarditis, seizures, cranial nerve lesions, paralysis, and coma. Death may occur from hyperpyrexia, massive bleeding, circulatory failure, splenic rupture, or a secondary infection.

Diagnosis

A positive diagnosis requires demonstration of the spirochetes in blood smears during febrile periods, using Wright's or Giemsa stain. *Borrelia* spirochetes may be harder to detect in later relapses, because their number in the blood declines. In such cases, injecting the patient's blood or tissue into a young rat and incubating the organism in the rat's blood for 1 to 10 days often facilitates spirochete identification.

In severe infection, spirochetes are found in the urine and cerebrospinal fluid. Other abnormal laboratory results include a white blood cell (WBC) count as high as 25,000/

mm³, and an increased lymphocyte count and erythrocyte sedimentation rate; however, the WBC count may be within normal limits. Because the *Borrelia* organism is a spirochete, relapsing fever may cause a false-positive test for syphilis.

Treatment

Oral tetracycline is the treatment of choice; it may be given I.V. if necessary and should continue for 4 to 5 days. In cases of tetracycline allergy or resistance, penicillin G may be administered as an alternative. However, neither drug should be given at the height of a severe febrile attack. If they are given, a Jarisch-Herxheimer reaction may occur, causing malaise, rigors, leukopenia, flushing, fever, tachycardia, rising respiratory rate, and hypotension. This reaction, which is caused by toxic by-products from massive spirochete destruction, can mimic septic shock and may prove fatal. Antimicrobial therapy should be postponed until the fever subsides. Until then, supportive therapy (consisting of parenteral fluids and electrolytes) should be given instead.

When neither tetracycline nor penicillin G controls relapsing fever, chloramphenicol may be given with caution. A complete blood count should be done regularly during treatment with chloramphenicol, because fatal granulocytopenia, thrombocytopenia, or even aplastic anemia may develop.

Special considerations

• During the initial evaluation period, obtain a complete history of the patient's travels.
• Throughout febrile periods, monitor vital signs, level of consciousness (LOC), and temperature every 4 hours. Watch for any signs of neurologic complications, such as decreasing LOC or seizures. To reduce fever, give tepid sponge baths and antipyretics.
• Maintain adequate fluid intake to prevent dehydration. Provide I.V. fluids. Measure intake and output accurately, especially if the patient is vomiting and has diarrhea.
• Administer antibiotics carefully. Document any hypersensitivity reactions (rash, fever, anaphylaxis), especially a Jarisch-Herxheimer reaction.
• Treat flushing, hypotension, or tachycardia with vasopressors or fluids.

• Look for symptoms of relapsing fever in family members and in others who may have been exposed to ticks or lice along with the victim.

• Use proper hand-washing technique, and teach it to the patient. Isolation is unnecessary because the disease isn't transmitted from person to person.

• Report all cases of louse- or tick-borne relapsing fever to the local public health department as required by law.

• To prevent relapsing fever, suggest to anyone traveling to tick-infested areas (Asia, northern and central Africa, South America) that they wear clothing that covers as much skin as possible. Sleeves and collars should be worn snugly and pant legs should be tucked into boots or socks.

Leprosy

A chronic, systemic infection, leprosy (Hansen's disease) is characterized by progressive cutaneous lesions. It's caused by *Mycobacterium leprae,* an acid-fast bacillus that attacks cutaneous tissue and peripheral nerves, producing skin lesions, anesthesia, infection, and deformities.

Leprosy occurs in three distinct forms:

• Lepromatous leprosy, the most serious type, causes damage to the upper respiratory tract, eyes, and testes, as well as the nerves and skin.

• Tuberculoid leprosy affects peripheral nerves and sometimes the surrounding skin, especially on the face, arms, legs, and buttocks.

• Borderline (dimorphous) leprosy has characteristics of both lepromatous and tuberculoid leprosies. Skin lesions in this type of leprosy are diffuse and poorly defined.

With timely and correct treatment, leprosy has a good prognosis and is rarely fatal. Untreated, however, it can cause severe disability. The lepromatous type may lead to blindness and deformities.

Causes

Contrary to popular belief, leprosy is not highly contagious. Rather, continuous, close contact is needed to transmit it. In fact, 9 out of 10 people have a natural immunity to it. Susceptibility appears highest during childhood and seems to decrease with age. Presumably, transmission occurs through airborne respiratory droplets containing *M. leprae* or by inoculation through skin breaks (with a contaminated hypodermic or tattoo needle, for example). The incubation period is unusually long – 6 months to 8 years.

Leprosy is most prevalent in the underdeveloped areas of Asia (especially India and China), Africa, South America, and the islands of the Caribbean and Pacific. About 15 million people worldwide suffer from this disease; approximately 4,000 are in the United States, mostly in California, Texas, Louisiana, Florida, New York, and Hawaii.

Signs and symptoms

M. leprae attacks the peripheral nervous system, especially the ulnar, radial, posterior-popliteal, anterior-tibial, and facial nerves. The central nervous system appears highly resistant. When the bacilli damage the skin's fine nerves, they cause anesthesia, anhidrosis, and dryness; if they attack a large nerve trunk, motor nerve damage, weakness, and pain occur, followed by peripheral anesthesia, muscle paralysis, or atrophy. In later stages, claw hand, foot drop, and ocular complications – such as corneal insensitivity and ulceration, conjunctivitis, photophobia, and blindness – can occur.

Injury, ulceration, infection, and disuse of the deformed parts cause scarring and contracture. Neurologic complications occur in both lepromatous and tuberculoid leprosies but are less extensive and develop more slowly in the lepromatous form. Lepromatous leprosy can invade tissue in all organs, but the organs generally remain functional.

Lepromatous and tuberculoid leprosies affect the skin in markedly different ways. In lepromatous disease, early lesions are multiple, symmetrical, and erythematous, sometimes appearing as macules or papules with smooth surfaces. Later, they enlarge and form plaques or nodules called lepromas on the earlobes, nose, eyebrows, and forehead. In advanced stages, *M. leprae* may infiltrate the entire skin surface. Lepromatous leprosy also causes loss of eyebrows, eyelashes, and sebaceous and sweat gland function; and, in advanced stages, conjunctival and scleral nodules. Upper respiratory lesions cause epistaxis, ulceration of the uvula and tonsils, septal perforation, and nasal collapse. Lepromatous leprosy can lead to hepatosplenomegaly and orchitis. Fingertips and toes deteriorate as bone resorption follows trauma and infection in these insensitive areas.

When tuberculoid leprosy affects the skin—sometimes its effect is strictly neural—it produces raised, large, erythematous plaques or macules with clearly defined borders. As they grow, they become rough, hairless, and hypopigmented, and leave anesthetic scars.

In borderline leprosy, skin lesions are numerous, but smaller, less anesthetic, and less sharply defined than tuberculoid lesions. Untreated, borderline leprosy may deteriorate into lepromatous disease.

Complications

Occasionally, acute episodes intensify leprosy's slowly progressing course. Erythema nodosum leprosum (ENL), seen in lepromatous leprosy, produces fever, malaise, lymphadenopathy, and painful red skin nodules, usually during antimicrobial treatment, although it may occur in untreated persons. In Mexico and other Central American countries, some patients with lepromatous disease develop Lucio's phenomenon, which produces generalized punched-out ulcers that may extend into muscle and fascia. Leprosy may also lead to tuberculosis, malaria, secondary bacterial infection of skin ulcers, and amyloidosis.

Diagnosis

Early clinical indications of skin lesions, and muscular and neurologic deficits are usually sufficiently diagnostic in patients from endemic areas. Biopsies of skin lesions are also diagnostic. Biopsies of peripheral nerves, or smears of the skin or of ulcerated mucous membranes, help confirm the diagnosis. Blood tests show increased erythrocyte sedimentation rate; decreased albumin, calcium, and cholesterol levels; and possibly anemia.

Treatment

Antimicrobial therapy consists of sulfones, primarily oral dapsone, which may cause hypersensitivity reactions. Hepatitis and exfoliative dermatitis, although uncommon, are especially dangerous reactions. If these reactions do occur, sulfone therapy should be stopped immediately.

Failure to respond to sulfone, respiratory involvement, or other complications require therapy such as rifampin in combination with clofazimine or ethionamide. Claw hand, wrist drop, or foot drop may require surgical correction.

When a patient's disease becomes inactive, as determined by the morphologic and bacterial index, treatment is discontinued according to the following schedule: tuberculoid—3 years; borderline—depends on the severity of the disease, but may be as long as 10 years; lepromatous—lifetime therapy. Since ENL is often considered a sign that the patient is responding to treatment, antimicrobial therapy should be continued. Thalidomide and clofazimine have been used successfully to treat ENL. Corticosteroids may also be given as part of ENL therapy.

Any patient suspected of having Hansen's disease may be referred to the Gillis W. Long Hansen's Disease Center in Carville, La., or to a regional center. At this international research and educational center, patients undergo diagnostic studies and treatment and are educated about their disease.

Special considerations

• Give antipyretics, analgesics, and sedatives as needed. Watch for ENL or Lucio's phenomenon.
• Tell the patient to cover coughs or sneezes with a paper tissue and to dispose of it properly. Take infection precautions when handling clothing or articles that have been in contact with open skin lesions.
• Patients with borderline or lepromatous leprosy may suffer eye complications, such as iridocyclitis and glaucoma. Decreased corneal sensation and lacrimation may also occur, requiring patients to use a tear substitute daily and protect their eyes to prevent corneal irritation and ulceration.
• Stress adequate nutrition and rest. Watch for fatigue, jaundice, and other signs of anemia and hepatitis.
• Tell the patient not to put too much weight on an anesthetized leg. Advise testing bathwater carefully to prevent scalding. To prevent ulcerations, suggest the use of sturdy footwear and soaking feet in warm water after any kind of exercise, even a short walk. Advise rubbing the feet with petroleum jelly, oil, or lanolin.
• For patients with deformities, rehabilitation employing a physiotherapist and plastic surgeon may be necessary. Teach the patient and help him with prescribed therapies.

Self-test questions

You can quickly review your comprehension of this chapter by answering the following questions. The correct answers to these questions and their rationales appear on pages 187 to 189.

Case history questions

Johnny Mills, age 9 months, lives in an inner city housing complex with his mother and four siblings, ages 3 to 7. One night, his mother brings him to the local hospital's emergency department. The initial examination reveals a spiking fever, chills, and a maculopapular rash. Physical manipulation elicits myalgia and arthralgia and reveals that Johnny is tachycardic and tachypneic. Meningococcemia is suspected.

1. Johnny is at particular risk for meningococcal infection because of his:
  a. sex.
  b. age.
  c. contact with school-age siblings.
  d. cramped living quarters.

2. Johnny probably contracted this infection through:
  a. inhalation of infected, aerosolized droplets.
  b. oral contact with a contaminated toy.
  c. ingestion of contaminated milk or water.
  d. the bite of an infected flea carried by the family dog.

3. Because a meningococcal infection is suspected, blood and cerebrospinal fluid cultures are obtained. Then Johnny should be:
  a. placed in strict isolation and treated symptomatically until cultures confirm the infecting organism and drug sensitivities.
  b. immediately started on large doses of ampicillin.
  c. treated with I.V. chloramphenicol.
  d. given minocycline to eradicate the infection.

4. Which of the following statements is true concerning the complications of fulminant meningococcemia?

    a. About 20% to 30% of patients progress from meningo-coccal bacteremia to fulminant meningococcemia.

    b. Intermittent fever, joint pain, and splenomegaly are characteristic symptoms of this disorder.

    c. Without prompt treatment, it results in death from respiratory or cardiac failure in 6 to 24 hours.

    d. Resultant tissue damage (possibly related to the effects of bacterial exotoxins) produces the fulminating symptoms.

Sixteen teenaged girls, all students at a local high school, are brought to the emergency department complaining of fever, abdominal pain, and severe diarrhea. Salmonellosis is suspected.

5. The patient history would focus primarily on the most common cause of salmonellosis, which is:

    a. contact with infected persons.

    b. fecal-oral spread associated with poor hand-washing technique.

    c. ingestion of contaminated foods, especially eggs and poultry.

    d. drinking from a contaminated water supply.

6. Which group has the greatest risk of contracting salmonellosis from sources that aren't clearly identifiable and exhibits recurrence after therapy?

    a. Infants

    b. Elderly people

    c. Patients with chronic degenerative diseases

    d. Patients with acquired immunodeficiency syndrome

7. Caregivers should use proper hand-washing technique, teach patients with salmonellosis the proper technique, and also observe:

    a. universal precautions.

    b. strict isolation.

    c. contact isolation.

    d. enteric precautions.

8. *Pseudomonas* infections may be recognized by their characteristic drainage, which is:
   a. milky white with a sour odor.
   b. yellow-green with a purulent odor.
   c. greenish blue with a sickly sweet odor.
   d. yellow-brown with a fecal odor.

9. Signs of septic shock include:
   a. oliguria and mental status changes.
   b. tachycardia with weak, thready pulse and hypotension.
   c. sudden fever and chills.
   d. hyperglycemia, thirst, and hyperpnea.

10. Which response is characteristic of infection with the *Haemophilus influenzae* bacillus?
   a. Lymph node tenderness leading to painful swelling and suppuration
   b. Acute suppurative inflammation
   c. A spasmodic, recurrent cough ending with a loud, crowing inspiration
   d. A thick, patchy, grayish green membrane over the mucosa of throat structures

CHAPTER 3

Viral Infections

Several hundred different viruses may infect humans and are spread chiefly by humans themselves. The diagnosis of viruses remains difficult. Viral diseases aren't susceptible to antibiotics, but sometimes antibiotics are used to prevent complications.

RESPIRATORY VIRUSES

Among the viral infections that affect the respiratory tract are the common cold, respiratory syncytial virus infection, parainfluenza, adenovirus infection, influenza, and hantavirus pulmonary syndrome.

Common cold

An acute, usually afebrile viral infection, the common cold causes inflammation of the upper respiratory tract. It accounts for more time lost from school or work than any other cause and is the most common infectious disorder. Although it's benign and self-limiting, it can lead to secondary bacterial infections.

Causes

The common cold is more prevalent in children than in adults; in adolescent boys than in girls; and in women than in men. In temperate zones, it occurs more often in the colder months; in the tropics, during the rainy season.

About 90% of colds stem from a viral infection of the upper respiratory passages and consequent mucous membrane inflammation; occasionally, colds result from mycoplasma. Over a hundred viruses can cause the common cold. Major offenders include rhinoviruses, coronaviruses, myxoviruses, adenoviruses, coxsackieviruses, and echoviruses.

Transmission occurs through airborne respiratory droplets, contact with contaminated objects, and hand-to-hand transmission. Children acquire new strains from their schoolmates and pass them on to family members. Fatigue or drafts don't increase susceptibility.

Signs and symptoms

After a 1- to 4-day incubation period, the common cold produces pharyngitis, nasal congestion, coryza, headache, and burning, watery eyes; there may be fever (in children), chills, myalgia, arthralgia, malaise, lethargy, and a hacking, nonproductive, or nocturnal cough.

As the cold progresses, clinical features develop more fully. After a day, symptoms include a feeling of fullness with a copious nasal discharge that often irritates the nose, adding to discomfort. About 3 days after onset, major signs diminish, but the "stuffed-up" feeling often persists for a week. Reinfection (with productive cough) is common, but complications (sinusitis, otitis media, pharyngitis, lower respiratory tract infection) are rare. A cold is communicable for 2 to 3 days after the onset of symptoms.

Diagnosis

No diagnostic test can isolate the specific organism responsible for the common cold. Consequently, diagnosis rests on the typically mild, localized, and afebrile upper respiratory tract symptoms. Despite infection, white blood count and differential are within normal limits.

Diagnosis must rule out allergic rhinitis, measles, rubella, and other disorders that produce similar early symptoms. A temperature higher than 100° F (37.8° C), severe malaise, anorexia, tachycardia, exudate on the tonsils or throat, petechiae, and tender lymph glands may point to more serious disorders and require additional diagnostic tests.

Treatment

The primary treatment—aspirin or acetaminophen, fluids, and rest—is purely symptomatic because the common cold has no cure. Aspirin eases myalgia and headache; fluids help loosen accumulated respiratory secretions and maintain hydration; and rest combats fatigue and weakness. In a child with a fever, acetaminophen is the drug of choice.

Decongestants can relieve congestion. Throat lozenges relieve soreness. Steam encourages expectoration. Nasal douching, sinus drainage, and antibiotics aren't necessary except in complications or chronic illness. Pure antitussives relieve severe coughs but are contraindicated with productive coughs, when cough suppression is harmful. The role of vitamin C remains controversial. In infants, saline nose drops and mucus aspiration with a bulb syringe may be beneficial.

Currently, no known measure can prevent the common cold. Vitamin therapy, interferon administration, and ultraviolet radiation are under investigation.

Special considerations

• Emphasize that antibiotics do not cure the common cold.
• Tell the patient to maintain bed rest during the first few days, to use a lubricant on his nostrils to decrease irritation, to relieve throat irritation with hard candy or cough drops, to increase fluid intake, and to eat light meals.
• Warm baths or heating pads can reduce aches and pains but won't hasten a cure. Suggest hot or cold steam vaporizers. Commercial expectorants are available, but their effectiveness is questionable.
• Advise against overuse of nose drops or sprays because these may cause rebound congestion.
• To help prevent colds, warn the patient to minimize contact with people who have colds. To avoid spreading colds, teach the patient to wash his hands often, to cover coughs and sneezes, and to avoid sharing towels and drinking glasses.

Respiratory syncytial virus infection

Respiratory syncytial virus (RSV) infection results from a subgroup of the myxoviruses resembling paramyxovirus. RSV is the leading cause of lower respiratory tract infections in infants and young children; it's the major cause of pneumonia, tracheobronchitis, and bronchiolitis in this age-group and a suspected cause of the fatal respiratory diseases of infancy.

Causes

Antibody titers seem to indicate that few children under age 4 escape contracting some form of RSV, even if it's mild. In fact, RSV is the only viral disease that has its maximum impact during the first few months of life (incidence of RSV bronchiolitis peaks at age 2 months).

This virus creates annual epidemics that occur during the late winter and early spring in temperate climates, and during the rainy season in the tropics. The organism is transmitted from person to person by respiratory secretions and has an incubation period of 4 to 5 days.

Reinfection is common, producing milder symptoms than the primary infection. School-age children, adolescents, and young adults with mild reinfections are probably the source of infection for infants and young children.

Signs and symptoms

Clinical features of RSV infection vary in severity, ranging from mild coldlike symptoms to bronchiolitis or bronchopneumonia and, in a few patients, severe, life-threatening lower respiratory tract infections. Generally, symptoms include coughing, wheezing, malaise, pharyngitis, dyspnea, and inflamed mucous membranes in the nose and throat.

Otitis media is a common complication of RSV in infants. RSV has also been identified in patients with a variety of central nervous system disorders, such as meningitis and myelitis.

Diagnosis

RSV infection is usually diagosed on the basis of clinical findings and epidemiologic information:

• Cultures of nasal and pharyngeal secretions may show RSV; however, the virus is very labile, so cultures aren't always reliable.
• Serum antibody titers may be elevated, but before 6 months of age, maternal antibodies may impair test results.
• Two recently developed serologic techniques are the indirect immunofluorescent and the enzyme-linked immunosorbent assay methods.
• Chest X-rays help detect pneumonia.

Treatment

Appropriate treatment aims to support respiratory function, maintain fluid balance, and relieve symptoms.

Special considerations

• Monitor respiratory status. Observe the rate and pattern; watch for nasal flaring or retraction, cyanosis, pallor, and dyspnea; listen or auscultate for wheezing, rhonchi, or other signs of respiratory distress. Monitor arterial blood gases and oxygen saturation.
• Maintain a patent airway, and be especially watchful when the patient has periods of acute dyspnea. Perform percussion, and provide drainage and suction when necessary. Use a croup tent to provide a high-humidity atmosphere. Placing the patient in a semi-Fowler's position may help prevent aspiration of secretions.
• Monitor intake and output carefully. Observe for signs of dehydration such as decreased skin turgor. Encourage the patient to drink plenty of high-calorie fluids. Administer I.V. fluids as needed.
• Promote bed rest.
• Hold and cuddle infants; talk to and play with toddlers. Offer suitable diversional activities to the child's condition and age. Foster parental visits and cuddling. Restrain child only as necessary.
• Impose oral secretion precautions. Enforce strict hand washing because RSV may be transmitted from fomites.
• Staff members with respiratory illnesses should not care for infants.

Parainfluenza

A general category of respiratory virus, parainfluenza refers to any of a group of respiratory illnesses caused by paramyxoviruses, a subgroup of the myxoviruses. Affecting both the upper and lower respiratory tracts, these self-limiting diseases resemble influenza but are milder and seldom fatal. Parainfluenza is rare among adults, but it's widespread among children. Incidence of parainfluenza in children rises in the winter and spring.

Causes

Parainfluenza is transmitted by direct contact or by inhalation of contaminated airborne droplets. Paramyxoviruses occur in four forms—Para 1 to 4—that are linked to several diseases: croup (Para 1, 2, 3), acute febrile respiratory illnesses (1, 2, 3), the common cold (1, 3, 4), pharyngitis (1, 3, 4), bronchitis (1, 3), and bronchopneumonia (1, 3). Para 3 ranks second to respiratory syncytial viruses as the most common infecting organism in lower respiratory tract infections in children. Para 4 rarely causes symptomatic infections in humans.

By age 8, most children demonstrate antibodies to Para 1 and Para 3. Most adults have antibodies to all four types as a result of childhood infections and subsequent multiple exposures. Reinfection is usually less severe and affects only the upper respiratory tract.

Signs and symptoms

After a short incubation period (usually 3 to 6 days), symptoms emerge that are similar to those of other respiratory diseases: sudden fever, nasal discharge, reddened throat (with little or no exudate), chills, and muscle pain. Bacterial complications are uncommon, but in infants and very young children, parainfluenza may lead to croup or laryngotracheobronchitis.

Diagnosis

Parainfluenza infections are usually clinically indistinguishable from similar viral infections. Isolation of the virus and serum antibody titers differentiate parainfluenza from other respiratory illness but are rarely done.

Treatment and special considerations   Parainfluenza may require no treatment or may require bed rest, antipyretics, analgesics, and antitussives, depending on the severity of the symptoms. Complications, such as croup and pneumonia, require appropriate treatment. No vaccine is effective against parainfluenza. Throughout this illness, monitor respiratory status and temperature, and ensure adequate fluid intake and rest.

Adenoviral infection

Adenoviruses cause acute, self-limiting, febrile infections, with inflammation of the respiratory or the ocular mucous membranes, or both.

Causes   Adenovirus has 35 known serotypes; it causes five major infections, all of which occur in epidemics. These organisms are common and can remain latent for years; they infect almost everyone early in life (though maternal antibodies offer some protection during the first 6 months of life).

Transmission of adenovirus can occur by direct inoculation into the eye, by the fecal-oral route (adenovirus may persist in the GI tract for years after infection), or by inhalation of an infected droplet. The incubation period is usually less than 1 week; acute illness lasts less than 5 days and can be followed by prolonged asymptomatic reinfection.

Signs and symptoms   Clinical features vary. (See *Major adenoviral infections,* page 102.)

Diagnosis   A definitive diagnosis requires isolation of the virus from respiratory or ocular secretions or fecal smears; during epidemics, however, typical symptoms alone can confirm diagnosis. Because adenoviral illnesses resolve rapidly, serum antibody titers aren't useful for diagnosis. Adenoviral diseases cause lymphocytosis in children. When they cause respiratory disease, chest X-rays may show pneumonitis.

Major adenoviral infections

DISEASE	AGE-GROUP	CLINICAL FEATURES
Acute febrile respiratory illness	Children	Nonspecific coldlike symptoms, similar to other viral respiratory illness: fever, pharyngitis, tracheitis, bronchitis, pneumonitis
Acute respiratory disease	Adults (usually military recruits)	Malaise, fever, chills, headache, pharyngitis, hoarseness, and dry cough
Viral pneumonia	Children and adults	Sudden onset of high fever, rapid infection of upper and lower respiratory tracts, skin rash, diarrhea, intestinal intussusception
Acute pharyngoconjunctival fever	Children (particularly after swimming in pools or lakes)	Spiking fever lasting several days, headache, pharyngitis, conjunctivitis, rhinitis, cervical adenitis
Acute follicular conjunctivitis	Adults	Unilateral tearing and mucoid discharge; later, milder symptoms in other eye
Epidemic keratoconjunctivitis	Adults	Unilateral or bilateral ocular redness and edema, preorbital swelling, local discomfort, superficial opacity of the cornea without ulceration
Hemorrhagic cystitis	Children (boys)	Hematuria, dysuria, urinary frequency

Treatment

Supportive treatment includes bed rest, antipyretics, and analgesics. Ocular infections may require corticosteroids and direct supervision by an ophthalmologist. Hospitalization is required in cases of pneumonia (in infants) to prevent death and in epidemic keratoconjunctivitis to prevent blindness.

Epidemic keratoconjunctivitis can be prevented by sterilization of ophthalmic instruments, adequate chlorination in swimming pools, and avoidance of swimming pools during epidemic keratoconjunctivitis outbreaks. Killed virus vaccine (not widely available) and a live oral virus vaccine can prevent adenoviral infection and are recommended for high-risk groups.

Special considerations

• During the acute illness, monitor respiratory status and intake and output.
• Give analgesics and antipyretics as needed.
• Stress the need for bed rest.

• To help minimize the incidence of adenoviral disease, instruct all patients in proper hand washing to reduce fecal-oral transmission.

Influenza

Also called the grippe or flu, influenza, an acute, highly contagious infection of the respiratory tract, results from three different types of *Myxovirus influenzae*. It occurs sporadically or in epidemics (usually during the colder months). Epidemics tend to peak within 2 to 3 weeks after initial cases and subside within a month.

Although influenza affects all age-groups, its incidence is highest in schoolchildren. However, its severity is greatest in the very young, elderly people, and those with chronic diseases. In these groups, influenza may even lead to death. The catastrophic pandemic of 1918 was responsible for an estimated 20 million deaths. The most recent pandemics— in 1957, 1968, and 1977—began in mainland China.

Causes

Transmission of influenza occurs through inhalation of a respiratory droplet from an infected person or by indirect contact, such as the use of a contaminated drinking glass. The influenza virus then invades the epithelia of the respiratory tract, causing inflammation and desquamation.

One of the remarkable features of the influenza virus is its capacity for antigenic variation. Such variation leads to infection by strains of the virus to which little or no immunologic resistance is present in the population at risk. Antigenic variation is characterized as *antigenic drift* (minor changes that occur yearly or every few years) and *antigenic shift* (major changes that lead to pandemics). Influenza viruses are classified into three groups:

• Type A, the most prevalent, strikes every year, with new serotypes causing epidemics every 3 years.
• Type B also strikes annually but causes epidemics only every 4 to 6 years.
• Type C is endemic and causes only sporadic cases.

Signs and symptoms

Following an incubation period of 24 to 48 hours, flu symptoms begin to appear: sudden onset of chills, temperature of 101° to 104° F (38.3° to 40° C), headache, malaise, myalgia (particularly in the back and limbs), a nonproductive cough, and, occasionally, laryngitis, hoarseness, conjunctivitis, rhinitis, and rhinorrhea. These symptoms usually subside in 3 to 5 days, but cough and weakness may persist. Fever is usually higher in children than in adults. Also, cervical adenopathy and croup are likely to be associated with influenza in children. In some patients (especially elderly people), lack of energy and easy fatigability may persist for several weeks.

Fever that persists longer than 3 to 5 days signals the onset of complications. The most common complication is pneumonia, which can be primary influenza viral pneumonia or secondary to bacterial infection. Influenza may also cause myositis, exacerbation of chronic obstructive pulmonary disease, Reye's syndrome, and, rarely, myocarditis, pericarditis, transverse myelitis, and encephalitis.

Diagnosis

At the beginning of an influenza epidemic, early cases are usually mistaken for other respiratory disorders. Because signs and symptoms are not pathognomonic, isolation of *M. influenzae* through inoculation of chicken embryos (with nasal secretions from infected patients) is essential at the first sign of an epidemic. In addition, nose and throat cultures and increased serum antibody titers help confirm this diagnosis.

After these measures confirm an influenza epidemic, diagnosis requires only observation of clinical signs and symptoms. Uncomplicated cases show decreased white blood cell counts with an increase in lymphocytes.

Treatment

In uncomplicated influenza, treatment includes bed rest, adequate fluid intake, aspirin or acetaminophen (the latter for children) to relieve fever and muscle pain, and guaifenesin or another expectorant to relieve nonproductive coughing. Prophylactic antibiotics aren't recommended because they have no effect on the influenza virus.

Amantadine (an antiviral agent) has proven to be effective in reducing the duration of signs and symptoms in influenza A infection. In influenza complicated by pneumonia, supportive care (liquid and electrolyte supplements, oxygen, assisted ventilation) and treatment of bacterial super-infection with appropriate antibiotics are necessary. No specific therapy exists for cardiac, central nervous system, or other complications.

Annual influenza inoculations may be given to high-risk patients and health care personnel. However, such vaccines are made from chicken embryos and must not be given to persons who are hypersensitive to eggs, feathers, or chickens. The vaccine administered is based on the previous year's virus and is usually about 75% effective.

Although the vaccine has not proved harmful to the fetus, it is not recommended for pregnant women, except those who are highly susceptible to influenza, such as women with chronic diseases. For people who are hypersensitive to eggs, amantadine is an effective alternative to the vaccine.

Special considerations

• Unless complications occur, influenza doesn't require hospitalization. Like treatment, patient care focuses on relief of symptoms.
• Advise the patient to use mouthwashes and increase his fluid intake. Warm baths or heating pads may relieve myalgia. Give him nonnarcotic analgesic-antipyretics as needed.
• Screen visitors to protect the patient from bacterial infection and visitors from influenza. Use respiratory precautions.
• Teach the patient proper disposal of paper tissues and proper hand-washing technique to prevent the virus from spreading.
• Watch for signs and symptoms of developing pneumonia, such as crackles, another temperature rise, or coughing accompanied by purulent or bloody sputum. Assist the patient in a gradual return to his normal activities.
• Educate patients about influenza immunizations. For high-risk patients and health care personnel, suggest annual inoculations at the start of the flu season (late autumn).
• Make all persons receiving the vaccine aware of possible adverse effects (discomfort at the vaccination site, fever, malaise and, rarely, Guillain-Barré syndrome).

Hantavirus pulmonary syndrome

Mainly occurring in the southwestern United States, but not confined to that area, hantavirus pulmonary syndrome was first reported in May 1993. The syndrome, which rapidly progresses from flulike symptoms to respiratory failure and, possibly, death, is known for its high mortality. The hantavirus strain that causes disease in Asia and Europe—mainly hemorrhagic fever and renal disease—is distinctly different from the one currently described in North America.

Causes

A member of the Bunyaviridae family, the genus *Hantavirus* (first isolated in 1977) is responsible for hantavirus pulmonary syndrome. Disease transmission is associated with exposure to infected rodents, the primary reservoir for this virus. Available data suggest that the deer mouse is the main source, but piñon mice, brush mice, and western chipmunks in close proximity to humans in rural areas are also sources. Hantavirus infections have been documented in people whose activities are associated with rodent contact, such as farming, hiking or camping in rodent-infested areas and occupying previously vacant cabins or rodent-infested dwellings.

Infected rodents manifest no apparent illness but shed the virus in feces, urine, and saliva. Human infection may occur from inhalation, ingestion (of contaminated food or water, for example), contact with rodent excrement, or rodent bites. Transmission from person to person or by mosquitos, fleas, or other arthropods hasn't been reported.

Signs and symptoms

Noncardiogenic pulmonary edema distinguishes the syndrome. Common chief complaints include myalgia, fever, headache, nausea and vomiting, and cough. Respiratory distress typically follows the onset of a cough. Fever, hypoxia and, in some patients, serious hypotension typify the hospital course.

Other signs and symptoms include a rising respiratory rate (28 breaths/minute or more) and an increased heart rate (120 beats/minute or more).

Screening for hantavirus pulmonary syndrome

Confirmed illness
The patient must have both of the following:
• at least one specimen (serum or tissue) available for laboratory testing to detect hantavirus infection
• in a patient with a compatible clinical illness, serologic evidence (presence of hantavirus-specific immunoglobulin M or rising titers of immunoglobulin G), polymerase chain reaction for hantavirus ribonucleic acid, or positive immunohistochemistry for hantavirus antigen.

Possible illness
The patient must have one of the following:
• a febrile illness (fever of at least 101° F [38.3° C]) in a previously healthy person with unexplained respiratory distress syndrome; or bilateral interstitial pulmonary infiltrates developing within 1 week of hospitalization, with respiratory compromise requiring supplemental oxygen
• an unexplained fatal respiratory illness

along with an autopsy demonstrating noncardiogenic pulmonary edema without an identifiable cause.

Absence of illness
For hantavirus pulmonary syndrome to be ruled out, the patient must have any of the following:
• a predisposing medical condition, such as severe pulmonary disease, solid tumors or hematologic cancers, congenital or acquired immunodeficiency, or other conditions, such as rheumatoid arthritis or organ transplantation, that require immunosuppressive therapy, such as corticosteroids or cytotoxic chemotherapy
• an acute illness that provides a likely explanation for the respiratory illness (for example, recent major trauma, burn, or surgery; recent seizures or history of aspiration; bacterial sepsis; another respiratory disorder such as respiratory syncytial virus in young children; influenza; or legionella pneumonia).

Diagnosis

• Despite ongoing efforts to identify clinical and laboratory features that distinguish hantavirus pulmonary syndrome from other infections with similar features, diagnosis currently is based on clinical suspicion along with a process of elimination developed by the Centers for Disease Control and Prevention (CDC) with the Council of State and Territorial Epidemiologists. (See *Screening for hantavirus pulmonary syndrome.*)

Note: The CDC and state health departments can perform definitive testing for hantavirus exposure and antibody formation.

• Laboratory tests usually reveal an elevated white blood cell count with a predominance of neutrophils, myeloid precursors, and atypical lymphocytes; elevated hematocrit; decreased platelet count; elevated partial thromboplastin time; and a normal fibrinogen level. Usually, laboratory findings

demonstrate only minimal abnormalities in renal function, with serum creatinine levels no higher than 2.5 mg/dl.
• Chest X-rays eventually show bilateral diffuse infiltrates in almost all patients (findings consistent with adult respiratory distress syndrome).

Treatment

Primarily supportive, treatment consists of maintaining adequate oxygenation, monitoring vital signs, and intervening to stabilize the patient's heart rate and blood pressure.

Drug therapy includes administering vasopressors, such as dopamine or epinephrine, for hypotension. Fluid volume replacement may also be ordered (with precautions not to overhydrate the patient).

Recent investigational drug therapy involves ongoing clinical trials with ribavirin.

Special considerations

• Assess the patient's respiratory status and arterial blood gas values often.
• Monitor serum electrolyte levels and correct imbalances as appropriate.
• Maintain a patent airway by suctioning. Ensure adequate humidification, and check ventilator settings frequently.
• In patients with hypoxemia, assess neurologic status frequently along with heart rate and blood pressure.
• Administer drug therapy and monitor the patient's response.
• Provide I.V. fluid therapy based on results of hemodynamic monitoring.
• Provide emotional support for the patient and his family.
• Report cases of hantavirus pulmonary syndrome to your state health department.
• Provide prevention guidelines. (Until more is known about hantavirus pulmonary syndrome, preventive measures currently focus on rodent control.)

RASH-PRODUCING VIRUSES

Some viral infections produce skin eruptions. They include varicella, rubella, rubeola, herpes simplex, herpes zoster, and variola.

Varicella

Also called chicken pox, varicella is a common, acute, and highly contagious infection caused by the herpesvirus varicella-zoster, the same virus that, in its latent stage, causes herpes zoster (shingles).

Causes

Chicken pox can occur at any age, but it's most common in 2- to 8-year-olds. Congenital varicella may affect infants whose mothers had acute infections in their first or early second trimester. Neonatal infection is rare, probably due to transient maternal immunity. Second attacks are also rare. This infection is transmitted by direct contact (primarily with respiratory secretions; less often, with skin lesions) and indirect contact (air waves). The incubation period lasts from 13 to 17 days. Chicken pox is probably communicable from 1 day before lesions erupt to 6 days after vesicles form (it's most contagious in the early stages of eruption of skin lesions).

Chicken pox occurs worldwide and is endemic in large cities. Outbreaks occur sporadically, usually in areas with large groups of susceptible children. It affects all races and both sexes equally. Seasonal distribution varies; in temperate areas, incidence is higher during late autumn, winter, and spring.

Most children recover completely. Potentially fatal complications may affect children receiving corticosteroids, antimetabolites, or other immunosuppressives, and those with leukemia, other neoplasms, or immunodeficiency disorders. Congenital and adult varicella may also have severe effects.

Signs and symptoms

Chicken pox produces distinctive signs and symptoms, notably a pruritic rash. During the prodromal phase, the patient has slight fever, malaise, and anorexia. Within 24 hours, the rash typically begins as crops of small, erythematous macules on the trunk or scalp that progress to papules and then clear vesicles on an erythematous base (the so-called "dewdrop on a rose petal"). The vesicles become cloudy and break easily; then scabs form. The rash spreads to the face and, rarely, to the extremities. New vesicles continue to appear for 3 or 4 days, so the rash contains a combination of red papules, vesicles, and scabs in various stages. Occasionally, chicken pox also produces shallow ulcers on mucous membranes of the mouth, conjunctivae, and genitalia.

Congenital varicella causes hypoplastic deformity and scarring of a limb, retarded growth, and central nervous system and eye manifestations. In progressive varicella, an immunocompromised patient will have lesions and a high fever for over 7 days.

Severe pruritus with this rash may provoke persistent scratching, which can lead to infection, scarring, impetigo, furuncles, and cellulitis. Rare complications include pneumonia, myocarditis, fulminating encephalitis (Reye's syndrome), bleeding disorders, arthritis, nephritis, hepatitis, and acute myositis.

Diagnosis

Positive diagnosis rests on characteristic clinical signs and usually doesn't require laboratory tests. However, the virus can be isolated from vesicular fluid within the first 3 or 4 days of the rash; Giemsa stain distinguishes varicella-zoster from vaccinia variola viruses. Serum contains antibodies 7 days after onset.

Treatment

Chicken pox calls for strict isolation until all the vesicles and most of the scabs disappear (usually for 1 week after the onset of the rash). Children can go back to school, however, if just a few scabs remain because, at this stage, chicken pox is no longer contagious. Congenital chicken pox requires no isolation.

Generally, treatment consists of local or systemic antipruritics: cool bicarbonate of soda baths, calamine lotion, or diphenhydramine or another antihistamine. Antibiotics are unnecessary unless bacterial infection develops. Salicylates are contraindicated because of their link with Reye's syndrome.

Susceptible patients may need special treatment. When given up to 72 hours after exposure to varicella, zoster immune globulin may provide passive immunity. Acyclovir may slow vesicle formation, speed skin healing, and control the systemic spread of infection.

Special considerations

- Teach the child and his family how to apply topical antipruritic medications correctly. Stress the importance of good hygiene.
- Tell the patient not to scratch the lesions. However, because the need to scratch may be overwhelming, parents should trim the child's fingernails or tie mittens on his hands.
- Warn parents to watch for and immediately report signs of complications. Severe skin pain and burning may indicate a serious secondary infection and require prompt medical attention.
- To help prevent chicken pox, don't admit a child exposed to chicken pox to a unit that contains children who receive immunosuppressive therapy or who have leukemia or immunodeficiency disorders. A vulnerable child who's been exposed to chicken pox should receive varicella-zoster immune globulin to lessen severity of the virus.

Rubella

Also called German measles, rubella is an acute, mildly contagious viral disease that produces a distinctive, 3-day rash and lymphadenopathy. It occurs most often among children ages 5 to 9, adolescents, and young adults. Worldwide in distribution, rubella flourishes during the spring (particularly in big cities) and epidemics occur sporadically. This disease is self-limiting, and the prognosis is excellent.

Causes

The rubella virus is transmitted through contact with the blood, urine, feces, or nasopharyngeal secretions of infected persons and possibly by contact with contaminated articles of clothing. Transplacental transmission, especially in the first trimester of pregnancy, can cause serious birth defects. Humans are the only known hosts for the rubella virus. The period of communicability lasts from about 10 days before until 5 days after the rash appears.

Signs and symptoms

In children, after an incubation period of from 16 to 18 days, an exanthematous, maculopapular rash erupts abruptly. In adolescents and adults, prodromal symptoms—headache, malaise, anorexia, low-grade fever, coryza, lymphadenopathy, and sometimes conjunctivitis—appear first. Suboccipital, postauricular, and postcervical lymph node enlargement is a hallmark of rubella.

Typically, the rubella rash begins on the face. This maculopapular eruption spreads rapidly, often covering the trunk and extremities within hours. Small, red, petechial macules on the soft palate (Forschheimer spots) may precede or accompany the rash. By the end of the second day, the facial rash begins to fade, but the rash on the trunk may be confluent and may be mistaken for scarlet fever. The rash continues to fade in the downward order in which it appeared. The rash generally disappears on the third day, but it may persist for 4 or 5 days—sometimes accompanied by mild coryza and conjunctivitis. The rapid appearance and disappearance of the rubella rash distinguishes it from rubeola.

Rubella can occur without a rash, but this is rare. Low-grade fever (99° to 101° F [37.2° to 38.3° C]) may accompany the rash, but it usually doesn't persist after the first day of the rash; rarely, temperature may reach 104° F (40° C).

Complications seldom occur in children with rubella, but when they do, they often appear as hemorrhagic problems, such as thrombocytopenia. Young women, however, often experience transient joint pain or arthritis, usually just as the rash is fading. Fever may then recur. These complications usually subside spontaneously within 5 to 30 days.

Diagnosis

The rubella rash, lymphadenopathy, other characteristic signs, and a history of exposure to infected persons usually permit clinical diagnosis without laboratory tests. However, cell cultures of the throat, blood, urine, and cerebrospinal fluid can confirm the virus' presence. Convalescent serum that shows a fourfold rise in antibody titers confirms the diagnosis.

Treatment

Because the rubella rash is self-limiting and only mildly pruritic, it doesn't require topical or systemic medication. Treatment consists of aspirin for fever and joint pain. Bed rest isn't necessary, but the patient should be isolated until the rash disappears.

Immunization with live virus vaccine RA 27/3, the only rubella vaccine available in the United States, is necessary for prevention and appears to be more immunogenic than previous vaccines. The rubella vaccine should be given with measles and mumps vaccines at age 15 months to decrease the cost and the number of injections needed.

Special considerations

• Make the patient with active rubella as comfortable as possible. Give children books to read or games to play to keep them occupied.

• Explain why respiratory isolation is necessary. Make sure the patient understands how important it is to avoid exposing pregnant women to this disease. (See *Understanding congenital rubella,* page 114.)

• Report confirmed cases of rubella to local public health officials.

• Know how to manage rubella immunization before giving the vaccine.

• Obtain a history of allergies, especially to neomycin. Having this allergy or a reaction to immunization in the past may determine whether the patient receives the vaccine.

• Ask women of childbearing age if they're pregnant. If they are or think they may be, *don't* give the vaccine. Warn women who receive rubella vaccine to use an effective means of birth control for at least 3 months after immunization.

• Give the vaccine at least 3 months after any administration of immune globulin or blood, which could have antibodies that neutralize the vaccine.

• Don't vaccinate any immunocompromised patients, patients with immunodeficiency diseases, or those receiving immunosuppressive, radiation, or corticosteroid therapy. Instead, administer immune serum globulin as ordered to prevent or reduce infection in susceptible patients.

Understanding congenital rubella

Congenital rubella is by far the most serious form of the disease. Intrauterine rubella infection, especially during the first trimester, can lead to spontaneous abortion or stillbirth, as well as single or multiple birth defects. (As a rule, the earlier the infection occurs during pregnancy, the greater the damage to the fetus.) The combination of cataracts, deafness, and cardiac disease composes the classic rubella syndrome. Low birth weight, microcephaly, and mental retardation are other common manifestations.

Prognosis depends on the particular malformations that occur. The overall mortality for rubella infants is 6%, but it's higher for babies born with thrombocytopenic purpura, congenital cardiac disease, or encephalitis.

Lifelong disease
Researchers now believe that congenital rubella can cause several more dis-orders, many of which don't appear until later in life. These include dental abnormalities, thrombocytopenic purpura, hemolytic and hypoplastic anemia, encephalitis, giant-cell hepatitis, seborrheic dermatitis, and diabetes mellitus. Indeed, it now appears that congenital rubella may be a lifelong disease. This theory is supported by the fact that the rubella virus has been isolated from urine 15 years after its acquisition in the uterus.

Care guidelines
Infants born with congenital rubella should be isolated immediately, because they excrete the virus for a period of from several months to a year after birth. Cataracts and cardiac defects may require surgery. Parents of affected children need emotional support and guidance in finding help from community resources and organizations.

• After giving the vaccine, observe for signs of anaphylaxis for at least 30 minutes. Keep epinephrine 1:1,000 handy.

• Warn about possible mild fever, slight rash, transient arthralgia (in adolescents), and arthritis (in elderly patients). Suggest aspirin or acetaminophen for fever.

• Advise the patient to apply warmth to the injection site for 24 hours after immunization (to help the body absorb the vaccine). If swelling persists after the initial 24 hours, suggest a cold compress to promote vasoconstriction and prevent antigenic cyst formation.

Rubeola

An acute, highly contagious paramyxovirus infection, rubeola (measles, morbilli) may be one of the most common and the most serious of all communicable childhood diseases. Use of the measles vaccine has reduced incidence of the disease during childhood; however, it's becoming more prevalent in adolescents and adults. (See *Administering measles vaccine*, page 116.) In the United States, the prognosis is usually excellent. However, measles is a major cause of death in children in underdeveloped countries.

Causes

Measles is spread by direct contact or by contaminated airborne respiratory droplets. The portal of entry is the upper respiratory tract. In temperate zones, incidence is highest in late winter and early spring. Before the availability of measles vaccine, epidemics occurred every 2 to 5 years in large urban areas.

Signs and symptoms

Incubation is from 10 to 14 days. Initial symptoms begin and greatest communicability occurs during a prodromal phase, about 11 days after exposure to the virus. This phase lasts from 4 to 5 days; symptoms include fever, photophobia, malaise, anorexia, conjunctivitis, coryza, hoarseness, and hacking cough.

At the end of the prodrome, Koplik's spots, the hallmark of the disease, appear. These spots look like tiny, bluish gray specks surrounded by a red halo. They appear on the oral mucosa opposite the molars and occasionally bleed.

About 5 days after Koplik's spots appear, temperature rises sharply, spots slough off, and a slightly pruritic rash appears. This characteristic rash starts as faint macules behind the ears and on the neck and cheeks. These macules become papular and erythematous, rapidly spreading over the entire face, neck, eyelids, arms, chest, back, abdomen, and thighs. When the rash reaches the feet (2 to 3 days later), it begins to fade in the same sequence it appeared, leaving a brownish discoloration that disappears in 7 to 10 days.

The disease climaxes 2 to 3 days after the rash appears and is marked by a temperature of 103° to 105° F (39.4° to

Administering measles vaccine

Generally, one bout of measles renders immunity (a second infection is extremely rare and may represent misdiagnosis); infants under age 4 months may be immune because of circulating maternal antibodies. Under normal conditions, measles vaccine isn't administered to children younger than age 15 months. However, during an epidemic, infants as young as 6 months may receive the vaccine; they must be reimmunized at age 15 months. An alternative approach calls for administration of gamma globulin to infants between ages 6 and 15 months who are likely to be exposed to measles.

Keep the following points in mind when administering measles vaccine:
• Warn the patient or his parents that possible adverse effects are anorexia, malaise, rash, mild thrombocytopenia or leukopenia, and fever. Advise that the vaccine may produce slight reactions, usually within 7 to 10 days.
• Ask the patient about known allergies, especially to neomycin (each dose contains a small amount). However, a patient who's allergic to eggs may receive the vaccine, because it contains only minimal amounts of albumin and yolk components.
• Avoid giving the vaccine to a pregnant woman (ask all women for the date of their last menstrual period). Warn female patients to avoid pregnancy for at least 3 months following vaccination.
• Don't vaccinate children with untreated tuberculosis, immunodeficiencies, leukemia or lymphoma, or those receiving immunosuppressives. If such children are exposed to the virus, recommend that they receive gamma globulin (gamma globulin won't prevent measles but will lessen its severity). Older unimmunized children who have been exposed to measles for more than 5 days may also require gamma globulin. Be sure to immunize them 3 months later.
• Delay vaccination for 8 to 12 weeks after administration of whole blood, plasma, or gamma globulin, because measles antibodies in these components may neutralize the vaccine.
• Watch for signs of anaphylaxis for 30 minutes after vaccination. Keep epinephrine 1:1,000 handy.
• Advise application of a warm compress to the vaccination site to facilitate absorption of the vaccine. If swelling occurs within 24 hours after vaccination, tell patient to apply cold compresses to promote vasoconstriction and to prevent antigenic cyst formation.

40.6° C), severe cough, puffy red eyes, and rhinorrhea. About 5 days after the rash appears, other symptoms disappear and communicability ends. Symptoms are usually mild in patients with partial immunity (conferred by administration of gamma globulin) or infants with transplacental antibodies. More severe symptoms and complications are more likely to develop in young infants, adolescents, adults, and immunocompromised patients than in young children.

Atypical measles may appear in patients who received the killed measles vaccine. These patients are acutely ill with a fever and a maculopapular rash that's most obvious in the arms and legs, or with pulmonary involvement and no skin lesions.

Severe infection may lead to secondary bacterial infection and to autoimmune reaction or organ invasion by the virus, resulting in otitis media, pneumonia, and encephalitis. Subacute sclerosing panencephalitis (SSPE), a rare and invariably fatal complication, may develop several years after measles. SSPE is less common in patients who have received the measles vaccine.

Diagnosis

Accurate diagnosis rests on distinctive clinical features, especially the pathognomonic Koplik's spots. Mild measles may resemble rubella, roseola infantum, enterovirus infection, toxoplasmosis, and drug eruptions; laboratory tests are required for a differential diagnosis. If necessary, measles virus may be isolated from the blood, nasopharyngeal secretions, and urine during the febrile period. Serum antibodies appear within 3 days after onset of the rash and reach peak titers 2 to 4 weeks later.

Treatment and special considerations

• Appropriate treatment for measles requires bed rest, relief of symptoms, and respiratory isolation throughout the communicable period. Vaporizers and a warm environment help reduce respiratory irritation, but cough preparations and antibiotics are generally ineffective; antipyretics can reduce fever. Therapy must also combat complications.
• Teach parents supportive measures, and stress the need for isolation, plenty of rest, and increased fluid intake.
• Advise parents to cope with photophobia by darkening the room or providing sunglasses, and to reduce fever with antipyretics and tepid sponge baths.
• Warn parents to watch for and report the early signs and symptoms of complications, such as encephalitis, otitis media, and pneumonia.

Herpes simplex

A recurrent viral infection, herpes simplex is caused by *Herpesvirus hominis* (HVH), a widespread infectious agent. Herpes type I, which is transmitted by oral and respiratory secretions, affects the skin and mucous membranes and commonly produces cold sores and fever blisters. Herpes type II primarily affects the genital area and is transmitted by sexual contact. However, cross-infection may result from urogenital sex.

Causes

About 85% of all HVH infections are subclinical. The others produce localized lesions and systemic reactions. After the first infection, a patient is a carrier susceptible to recurrent infections, which may be provoked by fever, menses, stress, heat, and cold. However, in recurrent infections, the patient usually has no constitutional signs and symptoms.

Primary HVH is the leading cause of childhood gingivostomatitis in children ages 1 to 3. It causes the most common form of nonepidemic encephalitis and is the second most common viral infection in pregnant women. It can pass to the fetus transplacentally and, in early pregnancy, may cause spontaneous abortion or premature birth. Herpes is equally common in males and females. Worldwide in distribution, it is most prevalent among children in lower socioeconomic groups who live in crowded environments. Saliva, skin lesions, purulent eye exudate, urine, and feces are potential sources of infection.

Signs and symptoms

In neonates, HVH symptoms usually appear a week or two after birth. They range from localized skin lesions to a disseminated infection of such organs as the liver, lungs, or brain. Common complications include seizures, mental retardation, blindness, chorioretinitis, deafness, microcephaly, diabetes insipidus, and spasticity. Up to 90% of infants with disseminated disease will die.

Primary infection in children may be generalized or localized and occurs after an incubation period of 2 to 12 days. After brief prodromal tingling and itching, localized infection causes typical primary lesions that erupt as vesicles on an erythematous base, eventually rupturing and leaving a painful ulcer, followed by a yellowish crust. Vesicles may form on any part of the oral mucosa, especially the tongue, gingiva, and cheeks. Healing begins 7 to 10 days after onset and is completed in 3 weeks.

Generalized infection begins with fever, pharyngitis, erythema, and edema. Vesicles occur with submaxillary lymphadenopathy, increased salivation, halitosis, anorexia, and fever of up to 105° F (40.6° C). Herpetic stomatitis may lead to severe dehydration in children. A generalized infection usually runs its course in 4 to 10 days. In this form, virus reactivation causes cold sores—single or grouped vesicles in and around the mouth.

Genital herpes usually affects adolescents and young adults. Typically painful, the initial attack produces fluid-filled vesicles that ulcerate and heal in 1 to 3 weeks. Fever, regional lymphadenopathy, and dysuria may also occur.

Usually, herpetic keratoconjunctivitis is unilateral and causes only local symptoms: conjunctivitis, regional adenopathy, blepharitis, and vesicles on the lid. Other ocular symptoms may be excessive lacrimation, edema, chemosis, photophobia, and purulent exudate.

Both types of HVH can cause acute sporadic encephalitis with an altered level of consciousness, personality changes, and seizures. Other effects may include olfactory and gustatory hallucinations and neurologic abnormalities such as aphasia.

Herpetic whitlow, an HVH finger infection, commonly affects nurses. First the finger tingles and then it becomes red, swollen, and painful. Vesicles with a red halo erupt and may ulcerate or coalesce. Other effects may include satellite vesicles, fever, chills, malaise, and a red streak up the arm.

Diagnosis

Typical lesions may suggest HVH infection. However, confirmation requires isolation of the virus from local lesions and histologic biopsy. A rise in antibodies and moderate leukocytosis may support the diagnosis.

Treatment

Generalized primary infection usually requires an analgesic-antipyretic to reduce fever and relieve pain. Anesthetic mouthwashes, such as viscous lidocaine, may reduce the pain of gingivostomatitis, enabling the patient to eat and preventing dehydration. Avoid alcohol-based mouthwashes. Drying agents, such as calamine lotion, ease the pain of labial or skin lesions. Avoid petroleum-based ointments, which promote viral spread and slow healing.

Refer patients with eye infections to an ophthalmologist. Topical corticosteroids are contraindicated in active infection, but idoxuridine, trifluridine, and vidarabine are effective.

A 5% acyclovir ointment may bring relief to patients with genital herpes or to immunosuppressed patients with HVH skin infections. Acyclovir I.V. helps treat more severe infections. Frequent prophylactic use of acyclovir in immunosuppressed transplant patients prevents disseminated disease.

Special considerations

• Teach patients with genital herpes to use warm compresses or take sitz baths several times a day; to use a drying agent, such as povidone-iodine solution; to increase fluid intake; and to avoid all sexual contact during the active stage.
• For pregnant women with HVH infection, recommend weekly viral cultures of the cervix and external genitalia starting at 32 weeks' gestation.
• Instruct patients with herpetic whitlow not to share towels or eating utensils. Educate staff members and other susceptible people about the risk of contagion. Abstain from direct patient care if you have herpetic whitlow.
• Tell patients with cold sores not to kiss infants or people with eczema. (Those with genital herpes pose no risk to infants if their hygiene is meticulous.)
• Patients with central nervous system infection alone need no isolation.

Herpes zoster

Also called shingles, herpes zoster is an acute unilateral and segmental inflammation of the dorsal root ganglia caused by infection with the herpesvirus varicella-zoster, which also causes chicken pox. This infection usually occurs in adults; it produces localized vesicular skin lesions confined to a dermatome, and severe neuralgic pain in peripheral areas innervated by the nerves arising in the inflamed root ganglia.

The prognosis is good unless the infection spreads to the brain. Eventually, most patients recover completely, except for possible scarring and, in corneal damage, visual impairment. Occasionally, neuralgia may persist for months or years.

Causes

Herpes zoster results from reactivation of varicella virus that has lain dormant in the cerebral ganglia (extramedullary ganglia of the cranial nerves) or the ganglia of posterior nerve roots since a previous episode of chicken pox. Exactly how or why this reactivation occurs isn't clear. Some believe that the virus multiplies as it's reactivated and that it's neutralized by antibodies remaining from the initial infection. But if effective antibodies aren't present, the virus continues to multiply in the ganglia, destroy the host neuron, and spread down the sensory nerves to the skin.

Herpes zoster occurs primarily in adults, especially those past age 50. It seldom recurs.

Signs and symptoms

Herpes zoster begins with fever and malaise. Within 2 to 4 days, severe deep pain, pruritus, and paresthesia or hyperesthesia develop, usually on the trunk and occasionally on the arms and legs in a dermatomal distribution. Pain may be continuous or intermittent and usually lasts from 1 to 4 weeks. Up to 2 weeks after the first symptoms, small, red, nodular skin lesions erupt on the painful areas. (These lesions commonly spread unilaterally around the thorax or vertically over the arms or legs.) Sometimes nodules don't appear at all, but when they do, they quickly become vesicles filled with clear fluid or pus. About 10 days after they appear, the vesicles dry and form scabs. When ruptured, such lesions often become infected and, in severe cases, may lead to the enlargement of regional lymph nodes; they may even become gangrenous. Intense pain may occur before the rash appears and after the scabs form.

Occasionally, herpes zoster involves the cranial nerves, especially the trigeminal and geniculate ganglia or the oculomotor nerve. Geniculate zoster may cause vesicle formation in the external auditory canal, ipsilateral facial palsy, hearing loss, dizziness, and loss of taste. Trigeminal ganglion involvement causes eye pain and, possibly, corneal and scleral damage and impaired vision. Rarely, oculomotor involvement causes conjunctivitis, extraocular weakness, ptosis, and paralytic mydriasis.

In rare cases, herpes zoster leads to generalized central nervous system infection, muscle atrophy, motor paralysis (usually transient), acute transverse myelitis, and ascending myelitis. More often, generalized infection causes acute retention of urine and unilateral paralysis of the diaphragm. In postherpetic neuralgia, a complication most common in the elderly, intractable neurologic pain may persist for years. Scars may be permanent.

Diagnosis

Herpes zoster diagnosis usually isn't possible until the characteristic skin lesions develop. Before then, the pain may mimic appendicitis, pleurisy, or other conditions. Examination of vesicular fluid and infected tissue shows eosinophilic intranuclear inclusions and varicella virus. Also, a lumbar puncture shows increased pressure; examination of cerebrospinal fluid shows increased protein levels and, possibly, pleocytosis. Differentiation of herpes zoster from localized herpes simplex requires staining antibodies from vesicular fluid and identification under fluorescent light.

Treatment

No specific treatment exists. The primary goal of supportive treatment is to relieve itching and neuralgic pain with calamine lotion or another antipruritic; aspirin, possibly with codeine or another analgesic; and, occasionally, collodion or tincture of benzoin applied to unbroken lesions. If bacteria have infected ruptured vesicles, the treatment plan usually includes an appropriate systemic antibiotic.

Trigeminal zoster with corneal involvement calls for instillation of idoxuridine ointment or another antiviral agent. To help a patient cope with the intractable pain of postherpetic neuralgia, the doctor may order a systemic corticosteroid—such as cortisone or, possibly, corticotropin—to reduce inflammation as well as tranquilizers, sedatives, or tricyclic antidepressants with phenothiazines. Acyclovir seems to stop progression of the rash and prevent visceral complications.

In immunocompromised patients—both children and adults—acyclovir may be administered I.V. The drug appears to prevent disseminated, life-threatening disease in some patients.

Special considerations

• Your care should emphasize keeping the patient comfortable, maintaining meticulous hygiene, and preventing infection. During the acute phase, adequate rest and supportive care can promote healing of lesions.

• If using calamine lotion, apply it liberally to the lesions. If lesions are severe and widespread, apply a wet dressing. Drying therapies, such as oxygen or air-loss bed and silver sulfadiazine ointment, may also be used.

• Instruct the patient to avoid scratching the lesions.

• If vesicles rupture, apply a cold compress.

• To ease the pain of oral lesions, suggest a soft toothbrush, a soft diet, and the use of a saline or bicarbonate mouthwash.

• To minimize neuralgic pain, never withhold or delay administration of analgesics. Give them exactly on schedule, because the pain of herpes zoster can be severe. In postherpetic neuralgia, consult a pain specialist to maximize pain relief without risking tolerance to the analgesic.

• Repeatedly reassure the patient that herpetic pain will eventually subside. Encourage diversionary and relaxing activities.

• Institute appropriate infection control precautions.

Variola

An acute, highly contagious infectious disease, variola (smallpox) was caused by the poxvirus *variola*. After a global eradication program, the World Health Organization pronounced smallpox eradicated on October 26, 1979, 2 years after the last naturally occurring case was reported in Somalia. Vaccination is no longer recommended, except for certain laboratory workers. The last known case in the United States was reported in 1949. Although naturally occurring smallpox has been eradicated, variola virus preserved in laboratories remains an unlikely source of infection.

Smallpox developed in three major forms: variola major (classic smallpox), which carried a high mortality; variola minor, a mild form that occurred in nonvaccinated persons and resulted from a less virulent strain; and varioloid, a mild variant of smallpox that occurred in previously vaccinated persons who had only partial immunity.

Causes

Smallpox affected people of all ages. In temperate zones, incidence was highest during the winter; in the tropics, during the hot, dry months. Smallpox was transmitted directly by respiratory droplets or dried scales of virus-containing lesions, or indirectly through contact with contaminated linens or other objects. Variola major was contagious from onset until after the last scab was shed.

Signs and symptoms

Characteristically, after an incubation period of 10 to 14 days, smallpox caused an abrupt onset of chills (and possibly seizures in children), high fever (temperature above 104° F [40° C]), headache, backache, severe malaise, vomiting (especially in children), marked prostration, and occasionally violent delirium, stupor, or coma. Two days after onset, symptoms became more severe, but by the third day the patient began to feel better.

However, he soon developed a sore throat and cough, and lesions appeared on the mucous membranes of the mouth, throat, and respiratory tract. Within days, skin lesions also appeared, progressing from macular to papular, vesicular, and pustular (pustules were as large as ⅓″ [8 mm] in diameter). During the pustular stage, the patient's temperature again rose, and early symptoms returned. By day 10, the pustules began to rupture; eventually, they dried and formed scabs. Symptoms finally subsided about 14 days after onset. Desquamation of the scabs took another 1 to 2 weeks, caused intense pruritus, and often left permanently disfiguring scars. In fatal cases, a diffuse dusky appearance came over the patient's face and upper chest. Death was the result of encephalitic manifestations, extensive bleeding from any or all orifices, or secondary bacterial infections.

Diagnosis

Smallpox was readily recognizable, especially during an epidemic or after known contact.

The most conclusive laboratory test was a culture of variola virus isolated from an aspirate of vesicles and pustules. Other laboratory tests included microscopic examination of smears from lesion scrapings, and complement fixation to detect the virus or its antibodies in the patient's blood.

Treatment and special considerations

• Initial treatment required hospitalization, with strict isolation, antimicrobial therapy to treat bacterial complications, and vigorous supportive measures.
• Symptomatic treatment of lesions with antipruritics was started during the pustular stage.
• Aspirin, codeine, or (as needed) morphine relieved pain.
• I.V. infusions and gastric tube feedings provided fluids, electrolytes, and calories, because pharyngeal lesions made swallowing difficult.

Roseola infantum

Also called exanthema subitum, roseola infantum is an acute, benign, presumably viral infection. It usually affects infants and young children (ages 6 months to 3 years). Characteristically, it first causes a high fever and then a rash that accompanies an abrupt drop to normal temperature.

Causes

Roseola affects boys and girls alike. It occurs year-round but is most prevalent in the spring and fall. Overt roseola, the most common exanthem in infants under age 2, affects 30% of all children; inapparent roseola (febrile illness without a rash) may affect the rest. The mode of transmission isn't known. Only rarely does an infected child transmit roseola to a sibling.

Signs and symptoms

After a 10- to 15-day incubation period, the infant with roseola develops an abruptly rising, unexplainable fever and, sometimes, seizures. Temperature peaks at 103° to 105° F (39.4° to 40.6° C) for 3 to 5 days, then drops suddenly. In the early febrile period, the infant may be anorexic, irritable, and listless but doesn't seem particularly ill. Simultaneously with

Incubation and duration of common rash-producing infections

INFECTION	INCUBATION (DAYS)	DURATION (DAYS)
Roseola	10 to 15	3 to 6
Varicella	10 to 14	7 to 14
Rubeola	13 to 17	5
Rubella	16 to 18	3
Herpes simplex	2 to 12	7 to 21

an abrupt drop in temperature, a maculopapular, nonpruritic rash develops, which blanches on pressure. The rash is profuse on the infant's trunk, arms, and neck and is mild on the face and legs. It fades within 24 hours. Although possible, complications are extremely rare.

Diagnosis

In roseola, diagnosis requires observation of the typical rash that appears about 48 hours after fever subsides. (See *Incubation and duration of common rash-producing infections.*)

Treatment

Because roseola is self-limiting, treatment is supportive and symptomatic: antipyretics to lower fever and, if necessary, anticonvulsants to relieve seizures.

Special considerations

• Teach parents how to lower their infant's fever by giving tepid baths, keeping him in lightweight clothes, and maintaining normal room temperature.
• Stress the need for adequate fluid intake.
• Tell parents that strict bed rest and isolation are unnecessary.
• Teach parents that a short febrile seizure will not cause brain damage. Explain that seizures will cease after fever subsides and that phenobarbital is likely to cause drowsiness; if it causes stupor, parents should call their doctor immediately.

ENTEROVIRUSES

Two of the syndromes caused by enteroviruses are herpangina and poliomyelitis.

Herpangina

This acute infection is caused by group A coxsackieviruses (usually types 1 through 10, 16, and 23) and, less commonly, by group B coxsackieviruses and echoviruses. The disease characteristically produces vesicular lesions on the mucous membranes of the soft palate, tonsillar pillars, and throat.

Causes

Because fecal-oral transfer is the main mode of transmission, herpangina usually affects children under age 10 (except neonates because of maternal antibodies). It occurs slightly more often in late summer and fall, and can be sporadic, endemic, or epidemic. Herpangina generally subsides in 4 to 7 days. (See *Enterovirus facts,* page 128.)

Signs and symptoms

After a 2- to 9-day incubation period, herpangina begins abruptly with a sore throat, pain on swallowing, a temperature of 100° to 104° F (37.8° to 40° C) that persists for 1 to 4 days and may cause seizures, headache, anorexia, vomiting, malaise, diarrhea, and pain in the stomach, back of the neck, legs, and arms. After this, up to 12 grayish white papulovesicles appear on the soft palate and, less frequently, on the tonsils, uvula, tongue, and larynx. These lesions grow from 1 to 2 mm in diameter to large, punched-out ulcers surrounded by small, inflamed margins.

Diagnosis

Characteristic oral lesions suggest this diagnosis; isolation of the virus from mouth washings or feces and elevated specific antibody titer confirm it. Other routine test results are normal except for slight leukocytosis.

Enterovirus facts

A genus of viruses, enteroviruses (polioviruses, coxsackieviruses, echoviruses) inhabit the GI tract. These viruses, among the smallest viruses that affect humans, include 3 known polioviruses, 23 group A coxsackieviruses, 6 group B coxsackieviruses, and 34 echoviruses. They usually infect humans as a result of ingestion of fecally contaminated ma-terial, causing a wide range of diseases (hand, foot, and mouth disease, aseptic meningitis, myocarditis, pericarditis, gastroenteritis, poliomyelitis). They can appear in the pharynx, feces, blood, cerebrospinal fluid, and central nervous system tissue. Enteroviral infections are more prevalent in the summer and fall.

Diagnosis requires distinguishing the mouth lesions in herpangina from those in streptococcal tonsillitis (no ulcers, lesions confined to tonsils).

Treatment

Appropriate treatment for herpangina is entirely symptomatic, emphasizing measures to reduce fever and prevent convulsions and possible dehydration. Herpangina doesn't require isolation or hospitalization.

Special considerations

• Tell parents that herpangina requires careful hand washing and sanitary disposal of excretions.
• Teach parents to give adequate fluids, enforce bed rest, and administer tepid sponge baths and antipyretics.

Poliomyelitis

An acute communicable disease, poliomyelitis (polio, infantile paralysis) is caused by the poliovirus and ranges in severity from inapparent infection to fatal paralytic illness. First recognized in 1840, poliomyelitis became epidemic in Norway and Sweden in 1905. Outbreaks reached pandemic proportions in Europe, North America, Australia, and New Zealand during the first half of this century. Incidence peaked during the 1940s and early 1950s and led to the development of the Salk vaccine. (See *Polio protection.*)

Polio protection

Dr. Jonas Salk's poliomyelitis vaccine, which became available in 1955, has been called one of the miracle drugs of modern medicine. The vaccine contains dead (formalin-inactivated) polioviruses that stimulate production of circulating antibodies in the human body. This vaccine so effectively eliminated poliomyelitis that today it's hard to appreciate how feared the disease once was.

Sabin vaccine
Today, the Sabin vaccine, which can be taken orally and is more than 90% effective, is the vaccine of choice in preventing poliomyelitis. The Sabin vaccine is available in trivalent and monovalent forms. Trivalent oral poliovirus vaccine (TOPV) contains live but weakened organisms of all three poliovirus serotypes in one solution. TOPV is generally preferred to the monovalent form, which contains only one viral type and is use-

ful only when the particular serotype is known.

Immunization guidelines
All infants should be immunized with the Sabin vaccine; pregnant women may be vaccinated without risk. However, because of the risk of contracting poliomyelitis from the vaccine, the vaccine is contraindicated in patients with immunodeficiency diseases, leukemia, or lymphoma and in those receiving corticosteroids, antimetabolites, other immunosuppressives, or radiation therapy. These patients are usually immunized with the Salk vaccine.

When possible, immunodeficient patients should avoid contact with family members who are receiving the Sabin vaccine for at least 2 weeks after vaccination. The Sabin vaccine is no longer routinely advised for adults unless they're at risk for exposure to polio or planning travel to endemic areas.

Minor polio outbreaks still occur, usually among non-immunized groups, as among the Amish of Pennsylvania in 1979. The disease strikes most often during the summer and fall. Once confined mainly to infants and children, poliomyelitis occurs more often today in people over age 15. Among children, it paralyzes boys most often; adults and girls are at greater risk for infection but not for paralysis.

The prognosis depends largely on the site affected. If the central nervous system (CNS) is spared, the prognosis is excellent. However, CNS infection can cause paralysis and death. The mortality for all types of poliomyelitis is 5% to 10%.

Causes

The poliovirus has three antigenically distinct serotypes — types I, II, and III — all of which cause poliomyelitis. These polioviruses are found worldwide and are transmitted from person to person by direct contact with infected oropharyngeal secretions or feces. The incubation period ranges from

5 to 35 days – 7 to 14 days on the average. The virus usually enters the body through the alimentary tract, multiplies in the oropharynx and lower intestinal tract, then spreads to regional lymph nodes and the blood. Factors that increase the probability of paralysis include pregnancy; old age; localized trauma, such as a recent tonsillectomy, tooth extraction, or inoculation; and unusual physical exertion at or just before clinical onset of poliomyelitis.

Signs and symptoms

Manifestations of poliomyelitis follow three basic patterns. Inapparent (subclinical) infections constitute 95% of all poliovirus infections. Abortive poliomyelitis (minor illness), which makes up between 4% and 8% of all cases, causes slight fever, malaise, headache, sore throat, inflamed pharynx, and vomiting. The patient usually recovers within 72 hours. Most inapparent and abortive cases of poliomyelitis go unnoticed.

Major poliomyelitis, however, involves the CNS and takes two forms: nonparalytic and paralytic. Children often show a biphasic course, in which the onset of major illness occurs after recovery from the minor illness stage. Nonparalytic poliomyelitis produces moderate fever, headache, vomiting, lethargy, irritability, and pains in the neck, back, arms, legs, and abdomen. It also causes muscle tenderness and spasms in the extensors of the neck and back, and sometimes in the hamstring and other muscles. (These spasms may be observed during maximum range-of-motion exercises.) Nonparalytic polio usually lasts about a week, with meningeal irritation persisting for about 2 weeks.

Paralytic poliomyelitis usually develops within 5 to 7 days of the onset of fever. The patient displays symptoms similar to those of nonparalytic poliomyelitis, with asymmetrical weakness of various muscles, loss of superficial and deep reflexes, paresthesia, hypersensitivity to touch, urine retention, constipation, and abdominal distention. The extent of paralysis depends on the level of the spinal cord lesions, which may be cervical, thoracic, or lumbar.

Resistance to neck flexion is characteristic in nonparalytic and paralytic poliomyelitis. The patient will "tripod" – extend his arms behind him for support – when he sits up. He'll display Hoyne's sign – his head will fall back when he is supine and his shoulders are elevated. From a supine position, he won't be able to raise his legs a full 90 degrees. Paralytic poliomyelitis also causes positive Kernig's and Brudzinski's signs.

When the disease affects the medulla of the brain, it's called bulbar paralytic poliomyelitis, which is the most perilous type. This form of poliomyelitis weakens the muscles supplied by the cranial nerves (particularly IX and X) and produces symptoms of encephalitis. Other symptoms include facial weakness, dysphagia, difficulty in chewing, inability to swallow or expel saliva, regurgitation of food through the nasal passages, and dyspnea, as well as abnormal respiratory rate, depth, and rhythm, which may lead to respiratory arrest. Fatal pulmonary edema and shock are possible.

Complications—many of which result from prolonged immobility and respiratory muscle failure—include hypertension, urinary tract infection, urolithiasis, atelectasis, pneumonia, myocarditis, cor pulmonale, skeletal and soft-tissue deformities, and paralytic ileus.

Diagnosis

In poliomyelitis, diagnosis requires isolation of the poliovirus from throat washings early in the disease, from stool specimens throughout the disease, and from cerebrospinal fluid (CSF) cultures in CNS infection. Coxsackievirus and echovirus infections must be ruled out. Convalescent serum antibody titers four times greater than acute titers support a diagnosis of poliomyelitis. Routine laboratory tests are usually within normal limits, though CSF pressure and protein levels may be slightly increased and white blood cell count elevated initially, mostly due to polymorphonuclear leukocytes, which constitute 50% to 90% of the total count. Thereafter, mononuclear cells constitute most of the diminished number of cells.

Treatment

Supportive treatment includes analgesics to ease headache, back pain, and leg spasms; morphine is contraindicated because of the danger of additional respiratory suppression. Moist heat applications may also reduce muscle spasm and pain.

Bed rest is necessary only until extreme discomfort subsides; in paralytic poliomyelitis, this may take a long time. Paralytic polio also requires long-term rehabilitation using physical therapy, braces, corrective shoes and, in some cases, orthopedic surgery.

Special considerations

• Your care must be comprehensive to help prevent complications and to assist polio patients physically and emotionally during their prolonged convalescence.
• Observe the patient carefully for signs of paralysis and other neurologic damage, which can occur rapidly.
• Maintain a patent airway, and watch for respiratory weakness and difficulty in swallowing. A tracheotomy is often done at the first sign of respiratory distress. Following this, the patient is then placed on a mechanical ventilator.
• Remember to reassure the patient that his breathing is being supported.
• Practice strict aseptic technique during suctioning. Be sure to use only sterile solutions to nebulize medications.
• Perform a brief neurologic assessment at least once a day, but don't demand any vigorous muscle activity. Encourage a return to mild activity as soon as the patient is able.
• Check blood pressure frequently, especially with bulbar poliomyelitis, which can cause hypertension or shock because of its effect on the brain stem.
• Watch for signs of fecal impaction (due to dehydration and intestinal inactivity). To prevent this, give sufficient fluids to ensure an adequate daily output of low-specific-gravity urine (1.5 to 2 liters/day for adults).
• Monitor the bedridden patient's food intake for an adequate, well-balanced diet. If tube feedings are required, give liquid baby foods, juices, lactose, and vitamins.
• To prevent pressure ulcers, provide good skin care, reposition the patient often, and keep the bed dry. Remember, muscle paralysis may cause bladder weakness or transient bladder paralysis.
• Apply high-top sneakers or use a foot board to prevent foot drop. To alleviate discomfort, use foam rubber pads and sandbags as needed and light splints.
• To control the spread of poliomyelitis, wash your hands thoroughly after contact with the patient, especially after contact with excretions. Instruct the ambulatory patient to do the same. (Only hospital personnel who have been vaccinated against poliomyelitis may have direct contact with the patient.)

• Provide emotional support to the patient and his family. Reassure the nonparalytic patient that his chances for recovery are good. Long-term support and encouragement are essential for maximum rehabilitation.

• When caring for a paralytic patient, help set up an interdisciplinary rehabilitation program. Such a program should include physical and occupational therapists, doctors, and, if necessary, a psychiatrist to help manage the emotional problems that develop in a patient suddenly facing severe physical disabilities.

ARBOVIRUS

Arboviruses are maintained in nature and transmitted to humans by mosquitoes and ticks.

Colorado tick fever

This benign infection that results from the Colorado tick fever virus, an arbovirus, is transmitted to humans by a hard-shelled wood tick called *Dermacentor andersoni.* The adult tick acquires the virus when it bites infected rodents, and remains permanently infective. Colorado tick fever occurs in the Rocky Mountain region of the United States, mostly in April and May at lower altitudes and in June and July at higher altitudes. Because of occupational or recreational exposure, it's more common in men than in women. Colorado tick fever apparently confers long-lasting immunity against reinfection.

Signs and symptoms

After a 3- to 6-day incubation period, Colorado tick fever begins abruptly with chills; a temperature of 104° F (40° C); severe aching of the back, arms, and legs; lethargy; and headache with eye movement. Photophobia, abdominal pain, nausea, and vomiting may occur. Rare effects include pete-chial or maculopapular rashes and central nervous system involvement. After several days, symptoms subside but re-turn within 2 to 3 days and continue for 3 more days before slowly disappearing. Complete recovery usually follows.

Diagnosis

A history of recent exposure to ticks and moderate to severe leukopenia, complement fixation tests, or virus isolation confirm the diagnosis.

Treatment

If possible, carefully remove the tick by grasping it with for-ceps or gloved fingers and pulling gently. Be careful not to crush the tick's body. Keep it for identification. Thoroughly wash the wound with soap and water. If the tick's head re-mains embedded, surgical removal is necessary. Give a tet-anus-diphtheria booster.

Special considerations

• Be alert for secondary infection.
• Monitor fluid and electrolyte balance, and provide replace-ment as needed.
• Reduce fever with antipyretics and tepid sponge baths.
• To prevent tick-borne infection, tell the patient to avoid tick bites by wearing protective clothing (long pants tucked into boots) and carefully checking his body and scalp for ticks several times a day whenever in infested areas.

MISCELLANEOUS VIRUSES

Included in this category are mumps, infectious mononucle-osis, rabies, cytomegalovirus infection, and Lassa fever.

Mumps

Also called infectious or epidemic parotitis, mumps is an acute viral disease caused by a paramyxovirus. It is most prevalent in children older than age 5 but younger than age 9. Infants less than age 1 seldom get this disease because of passive immunity from maternal antibodies. Peak incidence occurs during late winter and early spring. The prognosis for complete recovery is good, although mumps sometimes causes complications.

Causes

The mumps paramyxovirus is found in the saliva of an infected person and is transmitted by droplets or by direct contact. The virus is present in the saliva 6 days before to 9 days after onset of parotid gland swelling; the 48-hour period immediately preceding onset of swelling is probably the time of highest communicability. The incubation period ranges from 14 to 25 days (the average is 18). One attack of mumps (even if unilateral) almost always confers lifelong immunity.

Signs and symptoms

The clinical features of mumps vary widely. An estimated 30% of susceptible people have subclinical illness.

Mumps usually begins with prodromal symptoms that last for 24 hours and include myalgia, anorexia, malaise, headache, and low-grade fever, followed by an earache that's aggravated by chewing, parotid gland tenderness and swelling, a temperature of 101° to 104° F (38.3° to 40° C), and pain when chewing or when drinking sour or acidic liquids. Simultaneously with the swelling of the parotid gland or several days later, one or more of the other salivary glands may become swollen.

Complications include epididymo-orchitis and mumps meningitis. Epididymo-orchitis occurs in approximately 25% of postpubertal males who contract mumps, and produces abrupt onset of testicular swelling and tenderness, scrotal erythema, lower abdominal pain, nausea, vomiting, fever, and chills. Swelling and tenderness may last for several weeks; epididymitis may precede or accompany orchitis. In

50% of men with mumps-induced orchitis, the testicles show some atrophy, but sterility is extremely rare.

Mumps meningitis complicates mumps in 10% of patients and affects males three to five times more often than females. Symptoms include fever, meningeal irritation (nuchal rigidity, headache, and irritability), vomiting, drowsiness, and a cerebrospinal fluid lymphocyte count ranging from 500 to 2,000/mm³. Recovery is usually complete. Less common effects are pancreatitis, deafness, arthritis, myocarditis, encephalitis, pericarditis, oophoritis, and nephritis.

Diagnosis

In mumps, diagnosis is usually made after the characteristic signs and symptoms develop, especially parotid gland enlargement with a history of exposure to mumps. Serologic antibody testing can verify the diagnosis when parotid or other salivary gland enlargement is absent. If comparison between a blood specimen obtained during the acute phase of illness and another specimen obtained 3 weeks later shows a fourfold rise in antibody titer, the patient most likely had mumps.

Treatment

Appropriate treatment includes analgesics for pain, antipyretics for fever, and adequate fluid intake to prevent dehydration from fever and anorexia. If the patient can't swallow, consider I.V. liquid replacement.

Immunization within 24 hours of exposure may prevent or attenuate the actual disease. Immunity against mumps lasts at least 12 years.

Special considerations

• Stress the need for bed rest during the febrile period.
• Give analgesics and apply warm or cool compresses to the neck to relieve pain.
• Give antipyretics and tepid sponge baths for fever.
• To prevent dehydration, encourage the patient to drink fluids.
• To minimize pain and anorexia, advise the patient to avoid spicy, irritating foods and those that require a lot of chewing.
• During the acute phase, observe the patient closely for signs of central nervous system involvement, such as altered level of consciousness and nuchal rigidity.

• Because the mumps virus is present in the saliva throughout the course of the disease, respiratory isolation is recommended until symptoms subside.
• Emphasize the importance of routine immunization with live attenuated mumps virus (paramyxovirus) at age 15 months and for susceptible patients (especially males) who are approaching or are past puberty.
• Report all cases of mumps to local public health authorities.

Infectious mononucleosis

An acute infectious disease, infectious mononucleosis is caused by the Epstein-Barr virus (EBV), a member of the herpes group. It primarily affects young adults and children, although in children it's usually so mild that it's often overlooked. Characteristically, infectious mononucleosis produces fever, sore throat, and cervical lymphadenopathy (the hallmarks of the disease), as well as hepatic dysfunction, increased lymphocytes and monocytes, and development and persistence of heterophil antibodies. The prognosis is excellent, and major complications are uncommon.

Causes

Apparently, the reservoir of EBV is limited to humans. Infectious mononucleosis probably spreads by the oropharyngeal route, because about 80% of patients carry EBV in the throat during the acute infection and for an indefinite period afterward. It can also be transmitted by blood transfusion and has been reported after cardiac surgery as the post-perfusion syndrome. Infectious mononucleosis is probably contagious from before symptoms develop until the fever subsides and oropharyngeal lesions disappear.

Infectious mononucleosis is fairly common in the United States, Canada, and Europe, and both sexes are affected equally. Incidence varies seasonally among college students but not among the general population.

Signs and
symptoms

The symptoms of mononucleosis mimic those of many other infectious diseases, including hepatitis, rubella, and toxoplasmosis. Typically, after an incubation period of about 10 days in children and 30 to 50 days in adults, infectious mononucleosis produces prodromal symptoms, such as headache, malaise, and fatigue. After 3 to 5 days, patients typically develop a triad of symptoms: sore throat, cervical lymphadenopathy, and temperature fluctuations, with an evening peak of 101° to 102° F (38.3° to 38.9° C). Splenomegaly, hepatomegaly, stomatitis, exudative tonsillitis, or pharyngitis may also develop.

Sometimes, early in the illness, a maculopapular rash that resembles rubella develops; also, jaundice occurs in about 5% of patients. Major complications are rare but may include splenic rupture, aseptic meningitis, encephalitis, hemolytic anemia, autoimmune thrombocytopenic purpura, and Guillain-Barré syndrome. Symptoms usually subside about 6 to 10 days after onset of the disease but may persist for weeks.

Diagnosis

Physical examination demonstrating the clinical triad suggests infectious mononucleosis. The following abnormal laboratory results confirm it:
• Leukocyte count increases 10,000 to 20,000/mm³ during the second and third weeks of illness. Lymphocytes and monocytes account for 50% to 70% of the total white blood cell (WBC) count; 10% of the lymphocytes are atypical.
• Heterophil antibodies (agglutinins for sheep red blood cells) in serum drawn during the acute illness and at 3- to 4-week intervals rise to four times normal.
• Indirect immunofluorescence shows antibodies to EBV and cellular antigens. Such testing is usually more definitive than heterophil antibodies.
• Liver function studies are abnormal.

Treatment

Infectious mononucleosis resists prevention and antimicrobial treatment. Thus, therapy is essentially supportive: relief of symptoms, bed rest during the acute febrile period, and aspirin or another salicylate for headache and sore throat. If severe throat inflammation causes airway obstruction, steroids can be used to relieve swelling and avoid a tracheotomy. Splenic rupture, marked by sudden abdominal pain, requires splenectomy. About 20% of patients with infectious mononucleosis will also have streptococcal pharyngotonsillitis; these patients should receive antibiotic therapy for at least 10 days.

Special
considerations

• Because uncomplicated infectious mononucleosis doesn't require hospitalization, patient teaching is essential. Convalescence may take several weeks, usually until the patient's WBC count returns to normal.
• During the acute illness, stress the need for bed rest.
• If the patient is a student, tell him he may continue less demanding school assignments and see his friends but should avoid long, difficult projects until after recovery.
• To minimize throat discomfort, encourage the patient to drink milk shakes, fruit juices, and broths, and also to eat cool, bland foods. Advise the use of saline gargles and aspirin as needed.

Rabies

Usually transmitted by an animal bite, rabies (hydrophobia) is an acute central nervous system (CNS) infection caused by a ribonucleic acid virus. If symptoms occur, rabies is almost always fatal. Treatment soon after a bite, however, may prevent fatal CNS invasion.

Causes

Generally, the rabies virus is transmitted to a human through the bite of an infected animal that introduces the virus through the skin or mucous membrane. The virus begins to replicate in the striated muscle cells at the bite site. Then it spreads up the nerve to the CNS and replicates in the brain. Finally, it moves through the nerves into other tissues, including the salivary glands. Occasionally, airborne droplets and infected tissue transplants can transmit the virus.

If the bite is on the face, the risk of developing rabies is about 60%; on the upper extremities, 15% to 40%; and on the lower extremities, about 10%. In the United States, dog vaccinations have reduced rabies' transmission to humans. Wild animals, such as skunks, foxes, and bats, account for 70% of rabies cases.

Signs and symptoms

Typically, after an incubation period of 1 to 3 months, rabies produces local or radiating pain or burning, a sensation of cold, pruritus, and tingling at the bite site. It also produces prodromal symptoms, such as a slight fever (100° to 102° F [37.8° to 38.9° C]), malaise, headache, anorexia, nausea, sore throat, and a persistent loose cough. After this, the patient begins to show nervousness, anxiety, irritability, hyperesthesia, photophobia, sensitivity to loud noises, papillary dilation, tachycardia, shallow respirations, and excessive salivation, lacrimation, and perspiration.

About 2 to 10 days after onset of prodromal symptoms, a phase of excitation begins. It's characterized by agitation, marked restlessness, anxiety and apprehension, and cranial nerve dysfunction that causes ocular palsies, strabismus, asymmetrical papillary dilation or constriction, absence of corneal reflexes, weakness of facial muscles, and hoarseness. Severe systemic symptoms include tachycardia or bradycardia, cyclic respirations, urinary retention, and a temperature of about 103° F (39.4° C).

About 50% of affected patients exhibit hydrophobia (literally, "fear of water"), during which forceful, painful pharyngeal muscle spasms expel liquids from the mouth and cause dehydration and, possibly, apnea, cyanosis, and death. Difficulty swallowing causes frothy saliva to drool from the patient's mouth. Eventually, even the sight, mention, or thought of water causes uncontrollable pharyngeal muscle spasms and excessive salivation. Between episodes of excitation and hydrophobia, the patient commonly is cooperative and lucid.

After about 3 days, excitation and hydrophobia subside and the progressively paralytic, terminal phase of this illness begins. The patient experiences progressive, generalized, flaccid paralysis that ultimately leads to peripheral vascular collapse, coma, and death.

Diagnosis

Because rabies is fatal unless treated promptly, always suspect rabies in any person who suffers an unprovoked animal bite until you can prove otherwise. (See *First aid in animal bites.*)

First aid in animal bites

• Immediately wash the bite vigorously with soap and water for at least 10 minutes to remove the animal's saliva. Flush the wound with a viricidal agent, followed by a clear-water rinse.
• Apply a sterile dressing.
• If possible, don't suture the wound, and don't immediately stop the bleeding (unless it's massive) because blood flow helps to clean the wound.
• Question the patient about the bite. Ask if he provoked the animal (if so, chances are it's not rabid) and if he can identify it or its owner (the animal may be confined for observation).
• Consult local health authorities for treatment information.

Virus isolation from the patient's saliva or throat and examination of his blood for fluorescent rabies antibody (FRA) are considered the most diagnostic tests. Other results typically include elevated white blood cell count, with increased polymorphonuclear and large mononuclear cells, and elevated urinary glucose, acetone, and protein.

Confinement of the suspected animal for 10 days of observation by a veterinarian also helps support this diagnosis. If the animal appears rabid, it should be killed and its brain tissue tested for FRA and Negri bodies (oval or round masses that conclusively confirm rabies).

Treatment

In rabies, therapy consists of wound treatment and immunization as soon as possible after exposure. Thoroughly wash all bite wounds and scratches with soap and water. Check the patient's immunization status, and administer tetanus-diphtheria prophylaxis, if needed. Take measures to control bacterial infection as ordered. If the wound requires suturing, special treatment and suturing techniques must be used to allow proper wound drainage.

After rabies exposure, a patient who has not been immunized before must receive passive immunization with rabies immune globulin (Rig) and active immunization with human diploid cell vaccine (HDCV). If the patient has received HDCV before and has an adequate rabies antibody titer, he doesn't need Rig immunization, just an HDCV booster.

Special considerations	• When injecting rabies vaccine, rotate injection sites on the upper arm or thigh. Watch for and symptomatically treat redness, itching, pain, and tenderness at the injection site.

• When injecting rabies vaccine, rotate injection sites on the upper arm or thigh. Watch for and symptomatically treat redness, itching, pain, and tenderness at the injection site.

• Cooperate with public health authorities to determine the vaccination status of the animal. If the animal is proven rabid, help identify others at risk.

• If rabies develops, aggressive supportive care (even after onset of coma) can make probable death less agonizing.

• Monitor cardiac and pulmonary function continuously.

• Isolate the patient. Wear a gown, gloves, and protection for the eyes and mouth when handling saliva and articles contaminated with saliva. Take precautions to avoid being bitten by the patient during the excitation phase.

• Keep the room dark and quiet.

• Establish communication with the patient and his family. Provide psychological support to help them cope with the patient's symptoms and probable death.

• To help prevent rabies, stress the need for vaccination of household pets that may be exposed to rabid wild animals.

• Warn persons not to try to touch wild animals, especially if they appear ill or overly docile (a possible sign of rabies).

• Assist in the prophylactic administration of rabies vaccine to high-risk persons, such as farm workers, forest rangers, spelunkers (cave explorers), and veterinarians.

Cytomegalovirus infection

Highly host-specific, cytomegalovirus (CMV) infection is caused by the cytomegalovirus, which is a deoxyribonucleic acid, ether-sensitive virus belonging to the herpes family. (The disease is also called generalized salivary gland virus or cytomegalic inclusion disease [CID].) The disease occurs worldwide and is transmitted by human contact. About four out of five people over age 35 have been infected with cytomegalovirus, usually during childhood or early adulthood. In most of these people, the disease is so mild that it's overlooked. However, CMV infection during pregnancy can be hazardous to the fetus, possibly leading to stillbirth, brain damage, and other birth defects, or to severe neonatal illness.

Causes

CMV has been found in the saliva, urine, semen, breast milk, feces, blood, and vaginal and cervical secretions of infected persons.

The infection is usually transmitted through contact with infected secretions, which harbor the virus for months or even years. It may also be transmitted by sexual contact and can travel across the placenta causing a congenital infection. Immunosuppressed patients, especially those who have received transplanted organs, run a 90% chance of contracting CMV infection. Recipients of blood transfusions from donors with positive CMV antibodies are at some risk.

Signs and symptoms

CMV probably spreads through the body in lymphocytes or mononuclear cells to the lungs, liver, GI tract, eyes, and central nervous system, where it often produces inflammatory reactions.

Most patients with CMV infection have mild, nonspecific complaints, or none at all, even though antibody titers indicate infection. In these patients, the disease usually runs a self-limiting course. However, immunodeficient patients and those receiving immunosuppressives may develop pneumonia or other secondary infections. In patients with acquired immunodeficiency syndrome, disseminated CMV infection may cause chorioretinitis (resulting in blindness), colitis, or encephalitis. Infected infants ages 3 to 6 months usually appear asymptomatic but may develop hepatic dysfunction, hepatosplenomegaly, spider angiomas, pneumonitis, and lymphadenopathy.

Congenital CMV infection is seldom apparent at birth, though the infant's urine contains CMV. About 1% of all newborns have CMV.

The virus can cause brain damage that may not show up for months after birth. It can also produce a rapidly fatal neonatal illness characterized by jaundice, petechial rash, hepatosplenomegaly, thrombocytopenia, hemolytic anemia, microcephaly, psychomotor retardation, mental deficiency, and hearing loss. Occasionally, this form is rapidly fatal.

In some adults, CMV may cause cytomegalovirus mononucleosis, with 3 weeks or more of irregular, high fever.

C. Davis

Other findings may include a normal or elevated white blood cell (WBC) count, lymphocytosis, and increased atypical lymphocytes.

Diagnosis

Although virus isolation in urine is the most sensitive laboratory method, diagnosis can also rest on virus isolation from saliva, throat, cervix, WBC, and biopsy specimens.

Other laboratory tests support the diagnosis, including complement fixation studies, hemagglutination inhibition antibody tests, and, for congenital infections, indirect immunofluorescent tests for CMV immunoglobulin M antibody.

Treatment

Appropriate treatment aims to relieve symptoms and prevent complications. In the immunocompromised patient, CMV is treated with acyclovir, ganciclovir, and, possibly, foscarnet. Most important, parents of children with severe congenital CMV infection need support and counseling to help them cope with the possibility of brain damage or death.

Special considerations

• To help prevent CMV infection, warn immunocompromised patients and pregnant women to avoid exposure to confirmed or suspected CMV infection. (Maternal CMV infection can cause fetal abnormalities: hydrocephaly, microphthalmia, seizures, encephalitis, hepatosplenomegaly, hematologic changes, microcephaly, and blindness.)
• Urge patients with CMV infection to wash their hands thoroughly to prevent spreading it. It is especially important to stress this with young children.
• Be sure to observe universal precautions when handling body secretions.

Lassa fever

An epidemic hemorrhagic fever caused by the Lassa virus, Lassa fever is an extremely virulent arenavirus. As many as 100 cases occur annually in western Africa; the disease is rare in the United States. This highly fatal disorder kills 10%

to 50% of its victims, but those who survive its early stages usually recover and acquire immunity to secondary attacks.

Causes

A chronic infection in rodents, Lassa virus is transmitted to humans by contact with infected rodent urine, feces, and saliva. (This is the reason why Lassa fever sometimes strikes laboratory workers.) Then the virus enters the bloodstream, lymph vessels, and respiratory and digestive tracts. Following this, it multiplies in cells of the reticuloendothelial system. In the early stages of this illness, when the virus is in the throat, human transmission may occur through inhalation of infected droplets.

Signs and symptoms

After a 7- to 15-day incubation period, this disease produces a fever that persists for 2 to 3 weeks, exudative pharyngitis, oral ulcers, lymphadenopathy with swelling of the face and neck, purpura, conjunctivitis, and bradycardia. Severe infection may also cause hepatitis, myocarditis, pleural infection, encephalitis, and permanent unilateral or bilateral deafness. Virus multiplication in reticuloendothelial cells causes capillary lesions that lead to erythrocyte and platelet loss, mild to moderate thrombocytopenia (with a tendency to bleeding), and secondary bacterial infection. Capillary lesions also cause focal hemorrhage in the stomach, small intestine, kidneys, lungs, and brain and, possibly, hemorrhagic shock and peripheral vascular collapse.

Diagnosis

Isolation of the Lassa virus from throat washings, pleural fluid, or blood confirms the diagnosis. Recent travel to an endemic area and specific antibody titer support this diagnosis.

Treatment

Supportive treatment of Lassa fever includes administration of antibiotics (depending on the organism cultured) for secondary bacterial infection, I.V. colloids for shock, analgesics for pain, and antipyretics for fever. Infusion of immune plasma from patients who've recovered from Lassa fever may be useful in treatment, but test results on the benefits of this type of therapy are inconclusive.

Special considerations

• Carefully monitor fluid and electrolytes, vital signs, and intake and output. Watch for signs of infection or shock.

• Strict isolation is necessary for at least 3 weeks, until the patient's throat washings and urine are free of the virus.

• To prevent the spread of this contagious disease, carefully dispose of or disinfect all materials contaminated with the infected patient's urine, feces, respiratory secretions, or exudates. Watch known contacts closely for at least 3 weeks for signs of the disease.

• Provide good mouth care. Remember to clean the patient's mouth with a soft bristled brush to avoid irritating his mouth ulcers. Ask your hospital's dietary department to supply a soft, bland, nonirritating diet.

• Immediately report all cases of Lassa fever to the public health authorities in your area.

• Immediately contact the Viral Diseases Division of the Centers for Disease Control and Prevention in Atlanta to get specific guidelines for managing suspected or confirmed cases of Lassa fever.

Self-test questions

You can quickly review your comprehension of this chapter on viral infections by answering the following questions. The correct answers to these questions and their rationales appear on pages 189 and 190.

Case history
questions

Doctors and nurse practitioners in your community suspect and have reported a possible influenza epidemic, based on the large numbers of patients with typical signs and symptoms.

1. How would you confirm an epidemic and isolate the responsible influenza virus type?
   a. Observe clinical signs and symptoms.
   b. Obtain a white blood cell (WBC) count showing decreased totals with an increased percentage of lymphocytes.
   c. Inoculate chick embryos with the nasal secretions of infected patients.
   d. Confirm an increase in serum antibody titers.

2. Pandemic infection by a strain of influenza virus to which little or no immunologic resistance is present results from:
   a. antigenic drift.
   b. antigenic shift.
   c. type C infections.
   d. annual type A and B infections.

3. Which of the following groups has the highest incidence of influenza?
   a. Very young children
   b. School-age children
   c. Working adults
   d. Elderly people

4. Which of the following influenza signs may indicate complications if it persists for longer than 5 days?
   a. Fever
   b. Nonproductive cough
   c. Cervical adenopathy
   d. Lack of energy and easy fatigue

Your new patient has a febrile illness with unexplained adult respiratory distress syndrome (ARDS) and a preliminary diagnosis of hantavirus pulmonary syndrome.

5. You would expect this patient's history to reveal activities that had involved contact with infected:
   a. mosquitoes.
   b. fleas.
   c. cats.
   d. rodents.

6. What are the most common physical findings in hantavirus infections?
   a. Increased heart and respiratory rates
   b. Severe hypotension
   c. Pulmonary edema
   d. Headache and myalgias

7. Ninety-four percent of patients with hantavirus pulmonary syndrome develop signs consistent with ARDS, such as:
    a. air in the pleural space.
    b. patchy bilateral consolidation.
    c. upper lobe consolidation with bulging of fissures.
    d. bilateral diffuse infiltrates.

Additional questions

8. Which of the following viral infections accounts for more lost time from school or work than any other cause?
    a. Influenza
    b. Adenovirus infections
    c. Common cold
    d. Respiratory syncytial virus infection

9. How long should strict isolation for varicella last?
    a. Until all vesicles have scabbed over
    b. Until all scabs have disappeared
    c. Until new red papules cease to appear
    d. Until all vesicles and most scabs disappear

10. The most definitive laboratory test for infectious mononucleosis is:
    a. a WBC count showing typical leukocytosis with lymphocytes and monocytes accounting for 50% to 70% of the total count.
    b. abnormal liver function studies.
    c. heterophil antibodies that rise to four times normal.
    d. indirect immunofluorescence that shows antibodies to Epstein-Barr virus and cellular antigens.

CHAPTER 4

Fungal Infections

Caused by such fungi as yeasts and molds, mycotic diseases may be superficial or systemic. Candidiasis, cryptococcosis, histoplasmosis, coccidioidomycosis, and sporotrichosis are among prevalent mycotic diseases.

Candidiasis

Also called candidosis and moniliasis, candidiasis usually stems from a mild, superficial infection by the *Candida* genus. Most often, it infects the nails (onychomycosis), skin (diaper rash), or mucous membranes, especially the oropharynx (thrush), vagina (moniliasis), esophagus, and GI tract. Rarely, these fungi enter the bloodstream and invade the kidneys, lungs, endocardium, brain, or other structures, causing serious infections. Such systemic infection is most prevalent among drug abusers and patients already hospitalized, particularly diabetic and immunosuppressed patients. The prognosis varies, depending on the patient's resistance.

Causes

Most cases of *Candida* infection result from *Candida albicans*. Other infective strains include *C. parapsilosis, C. tropicalis,* and *C. guilliermondi.* These fungi are part of the normal flora of the GI tract, mouth, vagina, and skin. They cause infection when some change in the body permits their sudden proliferation: rising glucose levels from diabetes mellitus; lowered resistance from a disease such as a carcinoma, an immunosuppressive drug, radiation, aging, or human immunodeficiency virus (HIV) infection; or systemic introduction from I.V. or urinary catheters, drug abuse, total parenteral nutrition, or surgery.

However, the most common predisposing factor remains the use of broad-spectrum antibiotics, which decrease the number of normal flora and permit an increasing number of candidal organisms. In addition, the infant of a mother with vaginal moniliasis can contract oral thrush while passing through the birth canal.

The incidence of candidiasis is rising because of wider use of I.V. therapy and an increasing number of immunocompromised patients, especially those with HIV infection.

Signs and symptoms

Symptoms of superficial candidiasis correspond to the site of infection:

• Skin – scaly, erythematous, popular rash, sometimes covered with exudate, appearing below the breast, between fingers, and at the axillae, groin, and umbilicus. In diaper rash, papules appear at the edges of the rash.

• Nails – red, swollen, darkened nail bed; occasionally, purulent discharge and the separation of a pruritic nail from the nail bed

• Oropharyngeal mucosa (thrush) – cream-colored or bluish white, lacelike patches of exudate on the tongue, mouth, or pharynx that reveal bloody engorgement when scraped. They may swell, causing respiratory distress in infants and may be painful or cause a burning sensation in the throats and mouths of adults.

• Esophageal mucosa – dysphagia, retrosternal pain, regurgitation, and, occasionally, scales in the mouth and throat

• Vaginal mucosa – white or yellow discharge, with pruritus and local excoriation; white or gray raised patches on vaginal walls, with local inflammation; dyspareunia.

Systemic infection produces high, spiking fever, chills, hypotension, prostration, myalgias, arthralgias, and rash. Specific symptoms depend on the site of infection:

• Pulmonary – hemoptysis, cough, fever

• Renal – fever, flank pain, dysuria, hematuria, pyuria, cloudy urine

• Brain – headache, nuchal rigidity, seizures, focal neurologic deficits

• Endocardium – systolic or diastolic murmur, fever, chest pain, embolic phenomena

• Eye – endophthalmitis, blurred vision, orbital or periorbital pain, scotoma, and exudate.

Diagnosis

In superficial candidiasis, diagnosis depends on evidence of *Candida* on a Gram stain of skin, vaginal scrapings, pus, or sputum, or on skin scrapings prepared in potassium hydroxide solution. Systemic infections require obtaining a specimen for blood or tissue culture.

Treatment

First, treatment aims to improve the underlying condition that predisposes the patient to candidiasis, such as controlling diabetes or discontinuing antibiotic therapy and catheterization, if possible.

Nystatin is an effective antifungal for superficial candidiasis. Clotrimazole, fluconazole, ketoconazole, and miconazole are effective in mucous membrane and vaginal *Candida* infections. Ketoconazole or fluconazole is the treatment of choice for chronic candidiasis of the mucous membranes. Treatment for systemic infection consists of I.V. amphotericin B or fluconazole.

Special considerations

• Instruct a patient using nystatin solution to swish it around in his mouth for several minutes before he swallows the solution.
• Swab nystatin on the oral mucosa of an infant with thrush.
• Provide the patient with a nonirritating mouthwash to loosen tenacious secretions and a soft toothbrush to avoid irritation.
• Relieve the patient's mouth discomfort with a topical anesthetic, such as lidocaine, at least 1 hour before meals. (It may suppress the gag reflex and cause aspiration.)
• Provide a soft diet for the patient with severe dysphagia. Tell the patient with mild dysphagia to chew food thoroughly, and make sure he doesn't choke.
• Use cornstarch or dry padding in intertriginous areas of obese patients to prevent irritation.
• Note dates of insertion of I.V. catheters and replace them according to your hospital's policy to prevent phlebitis.
• Evaluate the patient with candidiasis for underlying causes such as diabetes mellitus. If the patient is receiving amphotericin B for systemic candidiasis, he may have severe chills, fever, anorexia, nausea, and vomiting. Premedicate with acetaminophen, antihistamines, or antiemetics to help reduce adverse reactions.

• Frequently check vital signs of patients with systemic infections. Provide appropriate supportive care. In patients with renal involvement, carefully monitor intake and output and check urine for blood and protein.

• Monitor high-risk patients daily, especially those receiving antibiotics, for patchy areas, irritation, sore throat, bleeding of mouth or gums, or other signs of superinfection. Check for vaginal discharge; record color and amount.

• Encourage women in their third trimester of pregnancy to be examined for vaginal candidiasis to protect their infants from infection at birth.

Cryptococcosis

Caused by the fungus *Cryptococcus neoformans*, cryptococcosis usually begins as an asymptomatic pulmonary infection but disseminates to extrapulmonary sites, usually to the central nervous system (CNS), but also to the skin, bones, prostate gland, liver, or kidneys.

With appropriate treatment, prognosis in pulmonary cryptococcosis is good. CNS infection, however, can be fatal, but treatment dramatically reduces mortality.

Causes

Transmission is through inhalation of *C. neoformans* in particles of dust contaminated by pigeon feces that harbor this organism. Therefore, cryptococcosis is primarily an urban infection. It is most prevalent in men, usually those between ages 30 and 60, and is rare in children.

Cryptococcosis is especially likely to develop in immunocompromised patients, such as those with Hodgkin's disease, sarcoidosis, leukemia, or lymphoma and those who are receiving immunosuppressive agents.

Currently, patients with acquired immunodeficiency syndrome (AIDS) are by far the most commonly affected group.

Signs and symptoms

Typically, pulmonary cryptococcosis is asymptomatic. Onset of CNS involvement is gradual (cryptococcal meningitis). The disorder causes progressively severe frontal and temporal headache, diplopia, blurred vision, dizziness, ataxia, aphasia, vomiting, tinnitus, memory changes, inappropriate behavior, irritability, psychotic symptoms, convulsions, and fever. If untreated, symptoms progress to coma and death, usually a result of cerebral edema or hydrocephalus. Complications include optic atrophy, ataxia, hydrocephalus, deafness, paralysis, chronic brain syndrome, and personality changes.

Skin involvement produces red facial papules and other skin abscesses, with or without ulcerations; bone involvement produces painful osseous lesions of the long bones, skull, spine, and joints.

Diagnosis

Although a routine chest X-ray showing a pulmonary lesion may point to pulmonary cryptococcosis, this infection usually escapes diagnosis until it disseminates. Firm diagnosis requires identification of *C. neoformans* by culture of sputum, urine, prostatic secretions, bone marrow aspirate or biopsy, or pleural biopsy, and, in CNS infection, by an India ink preparation of cerebrospinal fluid (CSF) and culture. Blood cultures are positive only in severe infection.

Supportive values include increased antigen titer in serum and CSF in disseminated infection; increased CSF pressure, protein, and white blood cell count in CNS infection; and moderately decreased CSF glucose in about half these patients. Diagnosis must rule out cancer and tuberculosis.

Treatment

The patient with pulmonary cryptococcosis will require close medical observation for a year after diagnosis. Treatment is unnecessary unless extrapulmonary lesions develop or pulmonary lesions progress.

Treatment of disseminated infection calls for I.V. amphotericin B or fluconazole. Patients with AIDS will also need long-term therapy, usually with oral fluconazole.

Special considerations

• Cryptococcosis doesn't require isolation.
• Check the patient's vital functions, and note any changes in mental status, orientation, pupillary response, and motor function.
• Watch for headache, vomiting, and nuchal rigidity.

• Before giving I.V. amphotericin B, check for phlebitis. In fuse slowly and dilute as required—rapid infusion may cause circulatory collapse.
• Before therapy, draw blood for a serum electrolyte analysi to determine baseline renal status.
• During drug therapy, watch for decreased urine output elevated blood urea nitrogen and creatinine levels, and hy pokalemia.
• Monitor results of complete blood count, urinalysis, and magnesium, potassium, and liver function tests. Ask the pa tient to report hearing loss, tinnitus, or dizziness.
• Give analgesics, antihistamines, and antiemetics for fever chills, nausea, and vomiting.
• Provide psychological support to help the patient cope with long-term hospitalization.

Aspergillosis

An opportunistic infection, aspergillosis is caused by fungi c the genus *Aspergillus*, usually *A. fumigatus, A. flavus,* and *A niger.* It occurs in four major forms: aspergilloma, which produces a fungus ball in the lungs (called a mycetoma); al lergic aspergillosis, a hypersensitive asthmatic reaction to aspergillus antigens; aspergillosis endophthalmitis, an infec tion of the anterior and posterior chambers of the eye tha can lead to blindness; and disseminated aspergillosis, an acute infection that produces septicemia, thrombosis, and infarction of virtually any organ, but especially the heart lungs, brain, and kidneys.

Aspergillus may cause infection of the ear (otomycosis) cornea (mycotic keratitis), and prosthetic heart valves (en docarditis); pneumonia (especially in persons receiving im munosuppressive drugs, such as antineoplastic agents o high-dose steroids); sinusitis; and brain abscesses.

The prognosis varies with each form. Occasionally, as pergilloma causes fatal hemoptysis.

Causes

Aspergillus is found worldwide, often in fermenting compost piles and damp hay. It's transmitted by inhalation of fungal spores or, in aspergillosis endophthalmitis, by the invasion of spores through a wound or other tissue injury. It's a common laboratory contaminant.

Aspergillus produces clinical infection only in persons who become especially vulnerable to it. Such vulnerability can result from excessive or prolonged use of antibiotics, glucocorticoids, or other immunosuppressive agents; from radiation; from such conditions as acquired immunodeficiency syndrome, Hodgkin's disease, leukemia, azotemia, alcoholism, sarcoidosis, bronchitis, or bronchiectasis; from organ transplantation; and, in aspergilloma, from tuberculosis or another cavitary lung disease.

Signs and symptoms

The incubation period in aspergillosis ranges from a few days to weeks. In aspergilloma, colonization of the bronchial tree with *Aspergillus* produces plugs and atelectasis and forms a tangled ball of hyphae (fungal filaments), fibrin, and exudate in a cavity left by a previous illness, such as tuberculosis. Characteristically, aspergilloma either causes no symptoms or mimics tuberculosis, causing a productive cough and purulent or blood-tinged sputum, dyspnea, empyema, and lung abscesses.

Allergic aspergillosis causes wheezing, dyspnea, cough with some sputum production, pleural pain, and fever. Aspergillosis endophthalmitis usually appears 2 to 3 weeks after an eye injury or surgery, and accounts for half of all cases of endophthalmitis. It causes clouded vision, eye pain, and reddened conjunctivae. Eventually, *Aspergillus* infects the anterior and posterior chambers, where it produces purulent exudate.

In disseminated aspergillosis, *Aspergillus* invades blood vessels and causes thrombosis, infarctions, and the typical signs of septicemia (chills, fever, hypotension, delirium), with azotemia, hematuria, urinary tract obstruction, headaches, seizures, bone pain and tenderness, and soft-tissue swelling. It's rapidly fatal.

Diagnosis

In patients with aspergilloma, a chest X-ray reveals a crescent-shaped radiolucency surrounding a circular mass, but this is not definitive for aspergillosis. In aspergillosis endophthalmitis, a history of ocular trauma or surgery and a culture or exudate showing *Aspergillus* is diagnostic. In allergic aspergillosis, sputum examination shows eosinophils. Culture of mouth scrapings or sputum showing *Aspergillus* is inconclusive, because even healthy persons harbor this fungus. In disseminated aspergillosis, culture and microscopic examination of affected tissue can confirm diagnosis, but this form is usually diagnosed at autopsy.

Treatment and special considerations

Aspergillosis doesn't require isolation. Treatment of aspergilloma necessitates local excision of the lesion and supportive therapy, such as chest physiotherapy and coughing, to improve pulmonary function. Allergic aspergillosis requires desensitization and, possibly, steroid therapy. Disseminated aspergillosis and aspergillosis endophthalmitis require a 2- to 3-week course of I.V. amphotericin B (as well as prompt cessation of immunosuppressive therapy) and possibly flucytosine. However, the disseminated form of aspergillosis often resists amphotericin B therapy and rapidly progresses to death.

Histoplasmosis

This fungal infection is caused by *Histoplasma capsulatum.* (Histoplasmosis is also called Ohio Valley disease, Central Mississippi Valley disease, Appalachian Mountain disease, and Darling's disease.) In the United States, histoplasmosis occurs in three forms: primary acute histoplasmosis, progressive disseminated histoplasmosis (acute disseminated or chronic disseminated disease), and chronic pulmonary (cavitary) histoplasmosis, which produces cavitations in the lung similar to those in pulmonary tuberculosis.

A fourth form, African histoplasmosis, occurs only in Africa and is caused by the fungus *Histoplasma capsulatum* var. *duboisii.*

Prognosis varies with each form. The primary acute disease is benign; the progressive disseminated disease is fatal in approximately 90% of patients; and without proper chemotherapy, chronic pulmonary histoplasmosis is fatal in 50% of patients within years.

Causes

H. capsulatum is found in the feces of birds and bats or in soil contaminated by their feces, such as that near roosts, chicken coops, and barns; in caves; or underneath bridges. Histoplasmosis occurs worldwide, especially in the temperate areas of Asia, Africa, Europe, and North and South America. In the United States, it's most prevalent in the central and eastern states, especially in the Mississippi and Ohio River Valleys.

Transmission is through inhalation of *H. capsulatum* or *H. duboisii* spores or through the invasion of spores after minor skin trauma. Probably because of occupational exposure, histoplasmosis is more common in adult males. Fatal disseminated disease, however, is more common in infants and elderly men.

The incubation period is from 5 to 18 days, although chronic pulmonary histoplasmosis may progress slowly for many years.

Signs and symptoms

Symptoms vary with each form of this disease. Primary acute histoplasmosis may be asymptomatic or may cause symptoms of a mild respiratory illness similar to a severe cold or influenza. Typical clinical effects may include fever, malaise, headache, myalgia, anorexia, cough, and chest pain.

Progressive disseminated histoplasmosis causes hepatosplenomegaly, general lymphadenopathy, anorexia, weight loss, fever, and possibly ulceration of the tongue, palate, epiglottis, and larynx, with resulting pain, hoarseness, and dysphagia. It may also cause endocarditis, meningitis, pericarditis, and adrenal insufficiency.

Chronic pulmonary histoplasmosis mimics pulmonary tuberculosis and causes a productive cough, dyspnea, and occasional hemoptysis. Eventually, it produces weight loss, extreme weakness, breathlessness, and cyanosis.

African histoplasmosis produces cutaneous nodules, papules, and ulcers; lymphadenopathy; lesions of the skull and long bones; and visceral involvement without pulmonary lesions.

Diagnosis

A history of exposure to contaminated soil in an endemic area, miliary calcification in the lung or spleen, and a positive histoplasmin skin test indicate exposure to histoplasmosis. Rising complement fixation and agglutination titers (more than 1:32) strongly suggest histoplasmosis.

The diagnosis of histoplasmosis requires a morphologic examination of tissue biopsy and culture of *H. capsulatum* from sputum in acute primary and chronic pulmonary histoplasmosis, and from bone marrow, lymph node, blood, and infection sites in disseminated histoplasmosis. However, cultures take several weeks to grow these organisms. Faster diagnosis is possible with stained biopsies using Gomori's stains (methenamine silver) or periodic acid-Schiff reaction. Findings must rule out tuberculosis and other diseases that produce similar symptoms.

The diagnosis of histoplasmosis caused by *H. duboisii* necessitates examination of tissue biopsy and culture of the affected site.

Treatment

In histoplasmosis, treatment consists of antifungal therapy, surgery, and supportive care. Antifungal therapy is most important. Except for asymptomatic primary acute histoplasmosis (which resolves spontaneously) and the African form, histoplasmosis requires high-dose or long-term (10-week) therapy with amphotericin B or fluconazole. For a patient who also has acquired immunodeficiency syndrome, lifelong therapy with fluconazole is indicated.

Supportive care usually includes oxygen for respiratory distress, glucocorticoids for adrenal insufficiency, and parenteral fluids for dysphagia due to oral or laryngeal ulcerations. Histoplasmosis doesn't require the patient to be isolated.

Special considerations

• Patient care is primarily supportive.
• Administer drugs and teach patients about possible adverse reactions. Because amphotericin B may cause chills, fever, nausea, and vomiting, give appropriate antipyretics, antihistamines, and antiemetics as needed.
• Patients with chronic pulmonary or disseminated histoplasmosis also need psychological support because of long-term hospitalization. As needed, refer to a social worker or

occupational therapist. Help parents of children with this disease arrange for a visiting teacher.
• To help prevent histoplasmosis, teach persons in endemic areas to watch for early signs of this infection and to seek treatment promptly. Instruct persons who risk occupational exposure to contaminated soil to wear face masks.

Blastomycosis

Also called North American blastomycosis or Gilchrist's disease, blastomycosis is caused by the yeastlike fungus *Blastomyces dermatitidis,* which usually infects the lungs and produces bronchopneumonia. Less frequently, this fungus may disseminate through the blood and cause osteomyelitis and central nervous system (CNS), skin, and genital disorders. Untreated blastomycosis is slowly progressive and usually fatal; however, spontaneous remissions occasionally occur. With antifungal drug therapy and supportive treatment, the prognosis for patients with blastomycosis is good.

Causes

Blastomycosis is generally found in North America (where *B. dermatitidis* normally inhabits the soil) and is endemic to the southeastern United States. Sporadic cases have also been reported in Africa. Blastomycosis usually infects men ages 30 to 50, but no occupational link has been found. *B. dermatitidis is* probably inhaled by people who are in close contact with the soil. The incubation period may range from weeks to months. (See *How blastomycosis progresses,* page 160.)

Signs and symptoms

Initial signs and symptoms of pulmonary blastomycosis mimic those of a viral upper respiratory infection. These findings typically include a dry, hacking, or productive cough (occasionally hemoptysis), pleuritic chest pain, fever, shaking chills, night sweats, malaise, anorexia, and weight loss.

Cutaneous blastomycosis causes small, painless, nonpruritic, and nondistinctive macules or papules on exposed

How blastomycosis progresses

Blastomycosis can follow one of several courses, ranging from asymptomatic pneumonia followed by recovery with no further developments to symptomatic pneumonia that progresses to pulmonary disease with extrapulmonary involvement. It also can pass through both acute and chronic stages. Use the flowchart below to trace the various courses the disease can take.

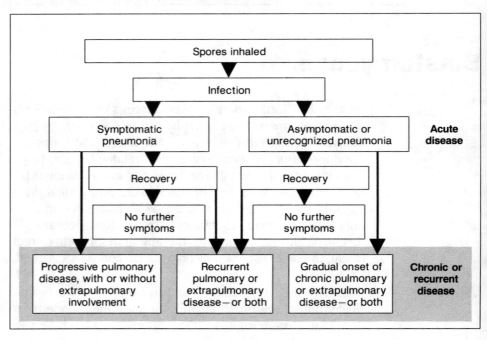

body parts. These lesions become raised and reddened, and occasionally progress to draining skin abscesses or fistulae.

Dissemination to the bone causes soft tissue swelling, tenderness, and warmth over bony lesions, which generally occur in the thoracic, lumbar, and sacral regions; long bones of the legs; and, in children, the skull.

Genital dissemination produces painful swelling of the testes, the epididymis, or the prostate; deep perineal pain; pyuria; and hematuria. CNS dissemination causes meningitis or cerebral abscesses that result in a decreased level of consciousness (LOC), lethargy, and change in mood or affect. Other dissemination may result in Addison's disease (adrenal insufficiency), pericarditis, and arthritis.

Diagnosis

The following tests are used to diagnose blastomycosis:
• *culture of B. dermatitidis* from skin lesions, pus, sputum, or pulmonary secretions
• microscopic examination of *tissue biopsy* from the skin or the lungs or of bronchial washings, sputum, or pus as appropriate
• *immunodiffusion testing,* which detects antibodies for the A and B antigen of blastomycosis
• *complement fixation testing.* (While such testing isn't conclusive, a high titer in extrapulmonary disease is a poor prognostic sign.)

In addition, suspected pulmonary blastomycosis requires a chest X-ray, which may show pulmonary infiltrates. Other abnormal laboratory findings include increased white blood cell count and erythrocyte sedimentation rate, slightly increased serum globulin, mild normochromic anemia, and, with bone lesions, increased alkaline phosphatase.

Treatment

All forms of blastomycosis respond to amphotericin B. Ketoconazole or fluconazole may be used as alternative agents. Patient care is mainly supportive.

Special considerations

• In severe pulmonary blastomycosis, check for hemoptysis. If the patient is febrile, provide a cool room and give tepid sponge baths.
• If blastomycosis causes joint pain or swelling, elevate the joint and apply heat. In CNS infection, watch the patient carefully for decreasing LOC and unequal pupillary response. In men with disseminated disease, watch for hematuria.
• Infuse I.V. amphotericin B slowly (too rapid infusion may cause circulatory collapse). During infusion, monitor vital signs (temperature may rise but should subside within 1 to 2 hours). Watch for decreased urine output and increased levels of blood urea nitrogen and creatinine, which may indicate renal toxicity. Monitor laboratory results for hypokalemia. Be alert for any hearing loss, tinnitus, or dizziness.
• To relieve adverse reactions to amphotericin B, give antiemetics and antipyretics.

Coccidioidomycosis

Caused by the fungus *Coccidioides immitis,* coccidioidomycosis is also called Valley fever or San Joaquin Valley fever.
The disorder occurs primarily as a respiratory infection, although generalized dissemination may occur. The primary
pulmonary form is usually self-limiting and rarely fatal. The
rare secondary (progressive, disseminated) form produces
abscesses throughout the body and carries a mortality of up
to 60%, even with treatment. Such dissemination is more
common in dark-skinned men, pregnant women, and patients who are receiving immunosuppressants.

Causes

Coccidioidomycosis is endemic to the southwestern United
States, especially between the San Joaquin Valley in California and southwestern Texas; it also is found in Mexico, Gua-
temala, Honduras, Venezuela, Colombia, Argentina, and
Paraguay. It may result from inhalation of *C. immitis* spores
found in the soil in these areas, or from inhalation of spores
from dressings or plaster casts of infected persons. It's most
prevalent during warm, dry months.

Because of population distribution and an occupational
link (it's common in migrant farm laborers), coccidioidomycosis generally strikes Filipino Americans, Mexican
Americans, Native Americans, and Blacks. In primary infection, the incubation period is from 1 to 4 weeks.

**Signs and
symptoms**

Primary coccidioidomycosis usually produces acute or subacute respiratory symptoms (dry cough, pleuritic chest pain,
pleural effusion), fever, sore throat, chills, malaise, headache, and an itchy macular rash. Occasionally, the sole
symptom is a fever that persists for weeks. From 3 days to
several weeks after onset, some patients, particularly Cau-
casian women, may develop tender red nodules (erythema
nodosum) on their legs, especially the shins, with joint pain
in the knees and ankles. Generally, the primary disease heals
spontaneously within a few weeks.

In rare cases, coccidioidomycosis disseminates to other
organs several weeks or months after the primary infection.
Disseminated coccidioidomycosis causes fever and ab-

scesses throughout the body, especially in skeletal, central nervous system (CNS), splenic, hepatic, renal, and subcutaneous tissues. Depending on the location of these abscesses, disseminated coccidioidomycosis may cause bone pain and meningitis. Chronic pulmonary cavitation, which can occur in both the primary and the disseminated forms, causes hemoptysis with or without chest pain.

Diagnosis

Typical clinical features and skin and serologic studies confirm this diagnosis. The primary form—and sometimes the disseminated form—produces a positive coccidioidin skin test. In the first week of illness, complement fixation for immunoglobulin G antibodies, or in the first month, positive serum precipitins (immunoglobulins) also establish this diagnosis. Examination or, more recently, immunodiffusion testing of sputum, pus from lesions, and a tissue biopsy may show *C. immitis* spores. The presence of antibodies in pleural and joint fluid and a rising serum or body fluid antibody titer indicate dissemination.

Other abnormal laboratory results include an increased white blood cell (WBC) count, eosinophilia, increased erythrocyte sedimentation rate, and a chest X-ray showing bilateral diffuse infiltrates.

In coccidioidal meningitis, examination of cerebrospinal fluid shows a WBC count increased to more than 500/mm³ (due primarily to mononuclear leukocytes), increased protein, and decreased glucose. Ventricular fluid obtained from the brain may contain complement fixation antibodies.

After diagnosis, the results of serial skin tests, blood cultures, and serologic testing may document the effectiveness of therapy.

Treatment

Usually, mild primary coccidioidomycosis requires only bed rest and relief of symptoms. Severe primary disease and dissemination, however, also require long-term I.V. infusion or, in CNS dissemination, intrathecal administration of amphotericin B, and, possibly, excision or drainage of lesions. Severe pulmonary lesions may require lobectomy. The antifungals miconazole and ketoconazole suppress *C. immitis* but do not eradicate it.

Special considerations
• Don't wash off the circle marked on the skin for serial skin tests because the circle aids in reading test results.
• In mild primary disease, encourage bed rest and adequate fluid intake. Record the amount and color of sputum. Watch for shortness of breath that may point to pleural effusion. In patients with arthralgia, provide analgesics.
• Coccidioidomycosis requires strict secretion precautions if the patient has draining lesions. "No touch" dressing technique and careful hand washing are essential.
• In CNS dissemination, monitor carefully for decreased level of consciousness or change in mood or affect.
• Before intrathecal administration of amphotericin B, explain the procedure to the patient, and reassure him that he'll receive analgesics before a lumbar puncture.
• If the patient is to receive amphotericin B intravenously, infuse it slowly because rapid infusion may cause circulatory collapse.
• During infusion, monitor vital signs (temperature may rise but should return to normal within 1 to 2 hours). Watch for decreased urinary output, and monitor laboratory results for elevated blood urea nitrogen and creatinine levels and hypokalemia.
• Tell the patient to immediately report hearing loss, tinnitus, dizziness, and all signs of toxicity.
• To ease adverse reactions to amphotericin B, give antiemetics and antipyretics.

Sporotrichosis

A chronic disease, sporotrichosis is caused by the fungus *Sporothrix schenckii*. It occurs in three forms: cutaneous lymphatic, which produces nodular erythematous primary lesions and secondary lesions along lymphatic channels; pulmonary, a rare form that produces a productive cough and pulmonary lesions; and disseminated, another rare form, which may cause arthritis or osteomyelitis.

The course of sporotrichosis is slow, prognosis is good, and fatalities are rare. However, untreated skin lesions may cause secondary bacterial infection.

Causes

S. schenckii is found in soil, wood, sphagnum moss, and decaying vegetation throughout the world. Because this fungus usually enters through broken skin (the pulmonary form through inhalation), sporotrichosis is more common in horticulturists, agricultural workers, and home gardeners. Perhaps because of occupational exposure, it's more prevalent in adult men than in women and children. The typical incubation period lasts from 1 week to 3 months.

Signs and symptoms

Cutaneous lymphatic sporotrichosis produces characteristic skin lesions, usually on the hands or fingers. Each lesion begins as a small, painless, movable subcutaneous nodule, but grows progressively larger, discolors, and eventually ulcerates. Later, additional lesions form along the adjacent lymph node chain.

Pulmonary sporotrichosis causes a productive cough, lung cavities and nodules, hilar adenopathy, pleural effusion, fibrosis, and the formation of a fungus ball. It's often associated with sarcoidosis and tuberculosis.

Disseminated sporotrichosis produces multifocal lesions that spread from the primary lesion in the skin or lungs. Onset is insidious. Typically, it causes weight loss, anorexia, synovial or bony lesions, and possibly arthritis or osteomyelitis.

Diagnosis

Typical clinical findings and culture of *S. schenckii* in sputum, pus, or bone drainage confirm this diagnosis. Histologic identification is difficult. Diagnosis must rule out tuberculosis, sarcoidosis, and, in patients with the disseminated form, bacterial osteomyelitis and neoplasm.

Treatment

Sporotrichosis doesn't require isolation. The cutaneous lymphatic form usually responds to application of a saturated solution of potassium iodide, which is generally continued for 1 to 2 months after the lesions have healed. Occasionally, cutaneous lesions must be excised or drained. The disseminated form responds to I.V. amphotericin B but may require several weeks of treatment. Local heat application relieves pain. Cavitary pulmonary lesions may require surgery.

Special
considerations

- Keep lesions clean, make the patient as comfortable as possible, and carefully dispose of contaminated dressings.
- Warn patients about possible adverse effects of drugs. Because amphotericin B may cause fever, chills, nausea, and vomiting, give antipyretics and antiemetics as necessary.
- To help prevent sporotrichosis, advise horticulturists and home gardeners to wear gloves while working.

Self-test questions

You can quickly review your comprehension of this chapter on fungal infections by answering the following questions. The correct answers to these questions appear on pages 225 to 227.

Case history
questions

Elsie Marks, a 58-year-old teacher with cancer, is currently receiving broad-spectrum I.V. antibiotics and immunosuppressive therapy. She has recently developed painful cream-colored pseudomembranous patches on her oral mucosa and a yellowish-white vaginal discharge with pruritus. Superficial candidiasis is diagnosed.

1. Which factor in Mrs. Marks' history is the most common predisposing factor for candidiasis?
- **a.** Aging
- **b.** Carcinoma
- **c.** Introduction of an I.V. catheter
- **d.** Use of broad-spectrum antibiotics

2. Which of the following factors places Mrs. Marks at high risk for systemic candidiasis?
- **a.** Hospitalization
- **b.** Immunosuppression
- **c.** Age
- **d.** Antibiotic therapy

3. Mrs. Marks should be closely observed for:
- **a.** high fever and chills.
- **b.** cough with hemoptysis.

    c. flank pain with dysuria and cloudy urine.
    d. headache and nuchal rigidity.

4. Treatment for systemic *Candida* infections consists of:
    a. clotrimazole.
    b. miconazole.
    c. ketaconazole or fluconazole.
    d. I.V. amphotericin B or fluconazole.

Albert Beaton, who works on a dairy farm, has been diagnosed with allergic aspergillosis, a hypersensitive reaction to Aspergillus *antigens.*

5. Which clinical findings would you expect Mr. Beaton to demonstrate?
    a. He would be asymptomatic.
    b. He would have a productive cough with purulent or blood-tinged sputum, dyspnea, empyema, and lung abscesses.
    c. He would exibit wheezing, dyspnea, cough with some sputum production, pleural pain, and fever.
    d. He would have reddened conjunctivae, eye pain, and clouded vision.

6. *Aspergillus* fungi spores are generally transmitted by:
    a. inhalation.
    b. wound invasion.
    c. ingestion.
    d. skin contamination.

7. Mr. Beaton's treatment will include:
    a. respiratory isolation.
    b. chest physiotherapy to improve pulmonary function.
    c. a 2- to 3-week course of I.V. amphotericin B.
    d. desensitization.

Additional questions

8. Cryptococcosis currently infects patients who have:
    a. sarcoidosis.
    b. leukemia.
    c. AIDS.
    d. Hodgkin's disease and lymphomas.

9. Histoplasmosis is more apt to occur as a fatal disseminated disease in:
   a. infants.
   b. adolescents.
   c. adult males.
   d. elderly females.

10. When administering I.V. amphotericin B to treat blastomycosis or other disseminated fungal infections, be careful to infuse it slowly because rapid infusion may cause:
   a. renal toxicity.
   b. circulatory collapse.
   c. ototoxicity.
   d. hyperpyrexia.

CHAPTER 5

Protozoal Infections

Such diseases as *Pneumocystis carinii* pneumonia, malaria, amebiasis, giardiasis, and toxoplasmosis result from minute but complex unicellular animals known as protozoa. These pathogens are known for their well-defined life cycles.

Pneumocystis carinii pneumonia

Because of its association with human immunodeficiency virus (HIV) infection, *Pneumocystis carinii* pneumonia (PCP), an opportunistic infection, has increased markedly in incidence since the 1980s. Before the advent of PCP prophylaxis, this disease was the first clue in about 60% of patients that HIV infection was present.

PCP strikes up to 90% of HIV-infected patients in North America. It can progress to pulmonary insufficiency and is the leading cause of death in these patients. Disseminated infection doesn't occur.

PCP also is associated with other immunocompromising conditions, including organ transplantation, leukemia, and lymphoma.

Causes

P. carinii, the cause of PCP, usually is classified as a protozoan, although some investigators consider it more closely related to fungi. The microorganism exists as a saprophyte in the lungs of humans and various animals. Part of the normal flora in most healthy people, *P. carinii* becomes an aggressive pathogen in the immunocompromised patient. Impaired cell-mediated (T-cell) immunity is thought to be more important than impaired humoral (B-cell) immunity in predisposing the patient to PCP, but the immune defects involved are poorly understood.

The microorganism invades the lungs bilaterally and multiplies extracellularly. As the infestation grows, alveoli fill with microorganisms and exudate, impairing gas exchange. The alveoli hypertrophy and thicken progressively, eventually leading to extensive consolidation.

The primary transmission route seems to be air, although the microorganism is already resident in most people. The incubation period probably lasts for 4 to 8 weeks.

Signs and symptoms

The patient typically has a history of an immunocompromising condition (such as HIV infection, leukemia, or lymphoma) or procedure (such as organ transplantation).

PCP begins insidiously with increasing shortness of breath and a nonproductive cough. Anorexia, fatigue, and weight loss may follow. Although the patient may have hypoxemia and hypercapnia, he may not exhibit significant symptoms. He may, however, have a low-grade, intermittent fever.

Other signs and symptoms include tachypnea, dyspnea, accessory muscle use for breathing, crackles (in about one-third of patients), and decreased breath sounds (in advanced pneumonia). Cyanosis may appear with acute illness; pulmonary consolidation develops later.

Diagnosis

• *Histologic studies* confirm *P. carinii* infection. In patients with HIV, initial examination of a first-morning sputum specimen (induced by inhaling an ultrasonically dispersed saline mist) may be sufficient; however, this technique usually is ineffective in patients without HIV.
• In all patients, *fiber-optic bronchoscopy* remains the most commonly used study to confirm PCP. Invasive procedures, such as transbronchial biopsy and open lung biopsy, are less commonly used.
• A *chest X-ray* may show slowly progressing, fluffy infiltrates and, occasionally, nodular lesions or a spontaneous pneumothorax, but these findings must be differentiated from findings in other types of pneumonia or adult respiratory distress syndrome.
• A *gallium scan* may show increased uptake over the lungs even when the chest X-ray appears relatively normal.

• In PCP, *arterial blood gas (ABG) studies* detect hypoxia and an increased A-a gradient.

Treatment

PCP may respond to drug therapy with co-trimoxazole or pentamidine isethionate. Moderate to severe PCP may also respond to trimetrexate glucuronate, a recently approved alternative treatment. Because of immune system impairment, many patients who also have HIV experience severe adverse reactions to drug therapy. These reactions include bone marrow suppression, thrush, fever, hepatotoxicity, and anaphylaxis. Nausea, vomiting, and rashes are common. Diphenhydramine may be used to treat the latter effects and leucovorin may reduce bone marrow suppression (and may be used prophylactically in HIV infection).

Pentamidine may be administered I.V. or in aerosol form. I.V. pentamidine may have severe toxic effects, whereas the inhaled form usually is well tolerated. However, inhaled pentamidine may not effectively reach the lung apices.

Supportive measures, such as oxygen therapy, mechanical ventilation, and maintaining adequate nutrition and fluid balance, are important adjunctive therapies.

Oral morphine sulfate solution may reduce the respiratory rate and anxiety, thereby enhancing oxygenation.

Special considerations

• Implement universal precautions.
• Frequently assess the patient's respiratory status, and monitor ABG levels. Administer oxygen therapy as needed.
• Encourage ambulation, deep-breathing exercises, and incentive spirometry to facilitate effective gas exchange.
• Administer antipyretics to relieve fever.
• Monitor intake and output and daily weight to evaluate fluid balance. Replace fluids.
• Give antimicrobial drugs as necessary. Never give pentamidine I.M. because it can cause pain and sterile abscesses. Administer the I.V. drug form slowly over 60 minutes to reduce the risk of hypotension.
• Monitor for adverse effects of antimicrobial drugs. If the patient is receiving co-trimoxazole, watch for nausea, vomiting, rash, bone marrow suppression, thrush, fever, hepatotoxicity, and anaphylaxis. If he's receiving pentamidine, watch for cardiac arrhythmias, hypotension, dizziness, azotemia, hypocalcemia, and hepatic disturbances.

• Provide diversional activities and adequate rest periods. Teach the patient energy conservation techniques as well.

• Supply nutritional supplements as needed. Encourage the patient to eat a high-calorie, protein-rich diet. Offer small, frequent meals if the patient cannot tolerate large amounts of food.

• Give emotional support and help the patient identify and use meaningful support systems.

• Instruct the patient about the medication regimen, especially about the adverse effects.

• If the patient will require oxygen therapy at home, explain that an oxygen concentrator may be most effective.

Malaria

An acute infectious disease, malaria is caused by protozoa of the genus *Plasmodium: P. falciparum, P. vivax, P. malariae,* and *P. ovale,* all of which are transmitted to humans by mosquito vectors. Falciparum malaria is the most severe form of the disease.

When treated, malaria is rarely fatal; untreated, it's fatal in 10% of victims, usually as a result of complications, such as disseminated intravascular coagulation (DIC). Untreated primary attacks last from a week to a month, or longer. Relapses are common and can recur sporadically for several years. Susceptibility to the disease is universal.

Causes

Malaria literally means "bad air" and for centuries was thought to result from the inhalation of swamp vapors. It is now known that malaria is transmitted by the bite of female *Anopheles* mosquitoes, which abound in humid, swampy areas. When an infected mosquito bites, it injects *Plasmodium* sporozoites into the wound. The infective sporozoites migrate by blood circulation to parenchymal cells of the liver; there they form cystlike structures containing thousands of merozoites.

Upon release, each merozoite invades an erythrocyte and feeds on hemoglobin. Eventually, the erythrocyte ruptures, releasing heme (malaria pigment), cell debris, and more merozoites that, unless destroyed by phagocytes, enter other erythrocytes. At this point, the infected person becomes a reservoir of malaria who infects any mosquito that feeds on him, thus beginning a new cycle of transmission. Hepatic parasites *(P. vivax, P. ovale,* and *P. malariae)* may persist for years in the liver and are responsible for the chronic carrier state. Because blood transfusions and street-drug paraphernalia can also spread malaria, drug addicts have a higher incidence of the disease.

Malaria is a tropical as well as a subtropical disease and is most prevalent in Asia, Africa, and Latin America. Incidence in the United States during the last 25 years has ranged from a high of 4,230 cases in 1970 (mainly among military personnel returning from Vietnam) to a low of 222 cases in 1973. The total number of reported cases of malaria in 1993 was 1,150. Typically, malaria transmission results from blood transfusions or the use of contaminated needles by drug addicts. (See *How to prevent malaria,* page 174.)

Signs and symptoms

After an incubation period of 12 to 30 days, malaria produces chills, fever, headache, and myalgia interspersed with periods of well-being (the hallmark of the benign form of malaria). Acute attacks (paroxysms) occur when erythrocytes rupture and have three stages:
• cold stage, lasting 1 to 2 hours, ranging from chills to extreme shaking
• hot stage, lasting 3 to 4 hours, characterized by a high fever (temperature up to 107° F [41.6° C])
• wet stage, lasting 2 to 4 hours, characterized by profuse sweating.

Paroxysms occur every 48 to 72 hours when malaria is caused by *P. malariae* and every 42 to 50 hours when malaria is caused by *P. vivax* or *P. ovale.* All three types have low levels of parasitosis and are self-limiting as a result of early acquired immunity.

Vivax and ovale malaria also produce hepatosplenomegaly. Hemolytic anemia is present in all but the mildest infections.

The most severe form of malaria is caused by *P. falciparum,* the only life-threatening strain. This species produces persistent high fever, orthostatic hypotension, and red blood

How to prevent malaria

• Drain, fill, and eliminate breeding areas of the *Anopheles* mosquito.
• Install screens in living and sleeping quarters in endemic areas.
• Use a residual insecticide on clothing and skin to prevent mosquito bites.
• Seek treatment for known cases.
• Question blood donors about a history of malaria or possible exposure to malaria. They *may* give blood if: they

haven't taken any antimalarial drugs and are asymptomatic after 6 months outside an endemic area; they were asymptomatic after treatment for malaria over 3 years ago; or they were asymptomatic after receiving malaria prophylaxis over 3 years ago.
• Seek prophylactic drug therapy before traveling to an endemic area.

---

cell (RBC) sludging that leads to capillary obstruction at various sites. Signs and symptoms of obstruction at these sites include the following:
• cerebral: hemiplegia, convulsions, delirium, coma
• pulmonary: coughing, hemoptysis
• splanchnic: vomiting, abdominal pain, diarrhea, melena
• renal: oliguria, anuria, uremia.

During blackwater fever (a complication of *P. falciparum* infection), massive intravascular hemolysis causes jaundice, hemoglobinuria, a tender and enlarged spleen, acute renal failure, and uremia. This dreaded complication is fatal in about 20% of patients.

Diagnosis

A history showing travel to endemic areas, recent blood transfusion, or drug abuse in a person with high fever of unknown origin strongly suggests malaria. But because symptoms of malaria mimic other diseases, unequivocal diagnosis depends on laboratory identification of the parasites in RBCs of peripheral blood smears.

The Centers For Disease Control and Prevention can identify donors responsible for transfusion malaria through indirect fluorescent serum antibody tests. These tests are unreliable in the acute phase, because antibodies can be undetectable for 2 weeks after onset.

Supplementary laboratory values that support this diagnosis include decreased hemoglobin, normal to decreased leukocyte count (as low as 3,000/mm^3), and protein and leukocytes in urine sediment. In falciparum malaria, serum values reflect DIC: reduced number of platelets (20,000 to 50,000/ mm³), prolonged prothrombin time (18 to 20 seconds), prolonged partial thromboplastin time (60 to 100 seconds), and decreased plasma fibrinogen.

Treatment

Malaria is best treated with oral chloroquine in all forms except chloroquine-resistant *P. falciparum.* Symptoms and parasitemia decrease within 24 hours after such therapy begins, and the patient usually recovers within 3 to 4 days. If the patient is comatose or vomiting frequently, chloroquine is given I.M. Rarely, toxic reactions include GI upset, pruritus, headache, and visual disturbances.

Malaria due to *P. falciparum,* which is resistant to chloroquine, requires treatment with oral quinine for 10 days, given concurrently with pyrimethamine and a sulfonamide, such as sulfadiazine. Relapses require the same treatment, or quinine alone, followed by tetracycline.

The only drug effective against the hepatic stage of the disease that is available in the United States is primaquine phosphate, given daily for 14 days. This drug can induce hemolytic anemia, especially in patients with a glucose-6-phosphate dehydrogenase deficiency.

For travelers spending less than 3 weeks in areas where malaria exists, weekly prophylaxis includes oral chloroquine beginning 2 weeks before and ending 6 weeks after the trip. Chloroquine and pyrimethamine with sulfadoxine may be ordered for those staying longer than 3 weeks, although combination treatment can have severe adverse effects. If the traveler isn't sensitive to either component of this drug, he may be given a single dose to take if he has a febrile episode. Any traveler who develops an acute febrile illness should seek prompt medical attention, regardless of prophylaxis taken. (See *Using antimalarial drugs,* page 176.)

Special considerations

• Obtain a detailed patient history, noting any recent travel, foreign residence, blood transfusion, or drug addiction. Record symptom pattern, fever, type of malaria, and any systemic signs.
• Assess the patient on admission and daily thereafter for fatigue, fever, orthostatic hypotension, disorientation, myalgia, and arthralgia. Enforce bed rest during periods of acute illness.

Using antimalarial drugs

Chloroquine
• Perform baseline and periodic ophthalmologic examinations. Be alert for blurred vision, increased sensitivity to light, and muscle weakness.
• Consider altering therapy if muscle weakness appears in a patient on long-term therapy.
• Monitor the patient for tinnitus.
• Caution the patient to avoid excessive exposure to the sun to prevent exacerbating drug-induced dermatoses.

Primaquine
• Give with meals or antacids.
• Stop administration if you observe a sudden fall in hemoglobin concentration or in erythrocyte or leukocyte count, or marked darkening of the urine, suggesting impending hemolytic reaction.

Pyrimethamine
• Administer with meals to minimize GI distress.
• Check blood counts (including platelets) twice a week. If signs of folic or folinic acid deficiency develop, reduce or discontinue dosage while the patient receives parenteral folinic acid until blood counts become normal.

Quinine
• Use with caution in the patient with a cardiovascular condition. Discontinue dosage if you see any signs of idiosyncrasy or toxicity, such as headache, epigastric distress, diarrhea, rashes, and pruritus, in a mild reaction; or delirium, convulsions, blindness, cardiovascular collapse, asthma, hemolytic anemia, and granulocytosis in a severe reaction.
• Monitor blood pressure often while administering quinine I.V. Rapid administration causes marked hypotension.

• Protect the patient from secondary bacterial infection by following proper hand-washing and aseptic techniques.
• Protect yourself by wearing gloves when handling blood or body fluids containing blood.
• Discard needles and syringes in an impervious container designated for incineration.
• Double-bag all contaminated linens and transport them according to hospital policy.
• To reduce fever, administer antipyretics. Document onset of fever and its duration and symptoms before and after episodes.
• Fluid balance is fragile, so keep a strict record of intake and output. Monitor I.V. fluids closely. Avoid fluid overload (especially with *P. falciparum*), because it can lead to pulmonary edema and the aggravation of cerebral symptoms.
• Observe blood chemistry levels for hyponatremia and increased blood urea nitrogen, creatinine, and bilirubin levels.

• Monitor urine output hourly, and maintain it at 40 to 60 ml/hour for an adult and at 15 to 30 ml/hour for a child.

• Watch for any decrease in urine output or the onset of hematuria as a possible sign of renal failure.

• Be prepared to do peritoneal dialysis for uremia caused by renal failure. For oliguria, administer furosemide or mannitol I.V.

• Slowly administer packed RBCs or whole blood while checking for crackles, tachycardia, and shortness of breath.

• If humidified oxygen is needed because of anemia, note the patient's response, particularly any changes in rate or character of respirations or improvement in mucous membrane color.

• Watch for signs of internal bleeding, such as tachycardia, hypotension, and pallor.

• Encourage frequent coughing and deep breathing, especially if the patient is on bed rest or has pulmonary complications. Record the amount and color of sputum.

• Watch for adverse effects of drug therapy, and take measures to relieve them.

• If the patient is comatose, make frequent, gentle changes in his position, and give passive range-of-motion exercises every 3 to 4 hours.

• If the patient is unconscious or disoriented, use restraints, as needed, and keep an airway or padded tongue blade available.

• Provide emotional support and reassurance, especially in critical illness. Explain the procedures and treatment to the patient and his family. Listen sympathetically, and answer questions clearly. Suggest that other family members be tested for malaria. Emphasize the need for follow-up care to check the effectiveness of treatment and to manage residual problems.

• Report all cases of malaria to the local public health authorities.

Amebiasis

Also called amebic dysentery, amebiasis is an acute or chronic protozoa infection caused by *Entamoeba histolytica*. This infection produces varying degrees of illness, from no symptoms at all or mild diarrhea to fulminating dysentery. Extraintestinal amebiasis can induce hepatic abscess and infections of the lungs, pleural cavity, pericardium, peritoneum, and, rarely, the brain.

Amebiasis occurs worldwide but is most common in the tropics, subtropics, and other areas with poor sanitation and health practices. Incidence in the United States averages between 1% and 3% but may be higher among homosexuals and institutionalized groups in whom fecal-oral contamination is common.

Prognosis is generally good, although complications — such as ameboma, intestinal stricture, hemorrhage or perforation, intussusception, or abscess — increase mortality. Brain abscess, a rare complication, is usually fatal.

Causes

E. histolytica exists in two forms: a cyst (which can survive outside the body), and a trophozoite (which can't survive outside the body). Transmission occurs through ingesting feces-contaminated food or water. The ingested cysts pass through the intestine, where digestive secretions break down the cysts and liberate the motile trophozoites within. The trophozoites multiply, and either invade and ulcerate the mucosa of the large intestine, or simply feed on intestinal bacteria. As the trophozoites are carried slowly toward the rectum, they are encysted and then excreted in feces. Man is the principal reservoir of infection.

Signs and symptoms

The clinical effects of amebiasis vary with the severity of the infection. Acute amebiasis causes a sudden high fever of 104° to 105° F (40° to 40.5° C) accompanied by chills and abdominal cramping; profuse, bloody diarrhea with tenesmus; and diffuse abdominal tenderness due to extensive rectosigmoid ulcers. Chronic amebiasis produces intermittent diarrhea that lasts for 1 to 4 weeks, and recurs several times a year. Such diarrhea produces 4 to 8 (or, in severe diarrhea, up to 18) foul-smelling mucus- and blood-tinged stools daily in a patient, along with a mild fever, vague abdominal cramps, possible weight loss, tenderness over the cecum and ascending colon, and occasionally hepatomegaly.

Amebic granuloma (ameboma), often mistaken for cancer, can be a complication of the chronic infection. Amebic granuloma produces blood and mucus in the stool and, when granulomatous tissue covers the entire circumference of the bowel, causes partial or complete obstruction.

Parasitic and bacterial invasion of the appendix may produce typical signs of subacute appendicitis (abdominal pain and tenderness). Occasionally, *E. histolytica* perforates the intestinal wall and spreads to the liver. When it perforates the liver and diaphragm, it spreads to the lungs, pleural cavity, peritoneum, and, rarely, the brain.

Diagnosis

Isolating *E. histolytica* (cysts and trophozoites) in fresh feces or aspirates from abscesses, ulcers, or tissue confirms acute amebic dysentery.

Diagnosis must distinguish between cancer and ameboma with X-rays, sigmoidoscopy, stool examination for amebae, and cecum palpation. In those with amebiasis, exploratory surgery is hazardous; it can lead to peritonitis, perforation, and pericecal abscess.

Other laboratory tests that support the diagnosis of amebiasis include:
• *indirect hemagglutination test* —positive with current or previous infection
• *complement fixation* —usually positive only during active disease
• *barium studies* —rule out nonamebic causes of diarrhea, such as polyps and cancer
• *sigmoidoscopy* —detects rectosigmoid ulceration; a biopsy may be helpful.

Patients with amebiasis shouldn't have preparatory enemas, because these may remove exudates and destroy the trophozoites, thus interfering with test results.

Treatment

Drugs used to treat amebiasis include metronidazole, an amebicide at intestinal and extraintestinal sites; emetine hydrochloride, also an amebicide at intestinal and extraintestinal sites, including the liver and lungs; iodoquinol (diiodohydroxyquin), an effective amebicide for asymptomatic carriers; chloroquine, for liver abscesses, not intestinal infections; and tetracycline (in combination with emetine hydrochloride, metronidazole, or paromomycin), which supports the antiamebic effect by destroying intestinal bacteria on which the amebae normally feed.

Special considerations

• Tell patients with amebiasis to avoid drinking alcohol when taking metronidazole. The combination may cause nausea, vomiting, and headache.

Giardiasis

An infection of the small bowel, giardiasis (also called enteritis and lambliasis) is caused by the symmetrical flagellate protozoan *Giardia lamblia*. A mild infection may not produce intestinal symptoms. In untreated giardiasis, symptoms wax and wane; with treatment, recovery is complete.

Causes

G. lamblia has two stages: the cystic stage and the trophozoite stage. Ingestion of *G. lamblia* cysts in fecally contaminated water or the fecal-oral transfer of cysts by an infected person results in giardiasis. When cysts enter the small bowel, they become trophozoites and attach themselves with their sucking disks to the bowel's epithelial surface. Following this, the trophozoites encyst again, travel down the colon, and are excreted. Unformed feces that pass quickly through the intestine may contain trophozoites as well as cysts.

Giardiasis occurs worldwide but is most common in developing countries and other areas where sanitation and hygiene are poor. In the United States, giardiasis is most common in travelers who've recently returned from endemic areas and in campers who drink unpurified water from contaminated streams. Probably because of frequent hand-to-mouth activity, children are more likely to become infected with *G. lamblia* than adults. In addition, hypogammaglobulinemia also appears to predispose persons to this disorder. Giardiasis doesn't confer immunity, so reinfections may occur.

Signs and symptoms

Attachment of *G. lamblia* to the intestinal lumen causes superficial mucosal invasion and destruction, inflammation, and irritation. All of these destructive effects decrease food transit time through the small intestine and result in malabsorption. Such malabsorption produces chronic GI complaints—such as abdominal cramps—and pale, loose, greasy, malodorous, and frequent stools (from 2 to 10 daily), with concurrent nausea. Stools may contain mucus but not pus or blood. Chronic giardiasis may produce fatigue and weight loss in addition to these typical signs and symptoms.

Diagnosis

Suspect giardiasis when travelers to endemic areas or campers who may have drunk unpurified water develop symptoms.

Actual diagnosis requires laboratory examination of a fresh stool specimen for cysts or examination of duodenal aspirate for trophozoites. A barium X-ray of the small bowel may show mucosal edema and barium segmentation. Diagnosis must also rule out other causes of diarrhea and malabsorption.

Treatment

Giardiasis responds readily to a 10-day course of metronidazole or a 7-day course of quinacrine and furazolidone P.O. Severe diarrhea may require parenteral fluid replacement to prevent dehydration if oral fluid intake is inadequate.

Special considerations

• Inform the patient receiving metronidazole of the expected adverse effects of this drug: commonly headache, anorexia, and nausea, and less commonly vomiting, diarrhea, and abdominal cramps.
• Warn against drinking alcoholic beverages because these may provoke a disulfiram-like reaction.
• If the patient is a woman, ask if she's pregnant, because metronidazole is contraindicated during pregnancy.
• When talking to family members and other suspected contacts, emphasize the importance of stool examinations for *G. lamblia* cysts.
• Hospitalization may be required. If so, apply enteric precautions. The patient will require a private room if he's a

child or an incontinent adult. When caring for such a patient, pay strict attention to hand washing, particularly after handling feces. Quickly dispose of fecal material. (Normal sewage systems can remove and process infected feces adequately.)

• Teach good personal hygiene, particularly proper hand-washing technique.

• To help prevent giardiasis, warn travelers to endemic areas not to drink water or eat uncooked and unpeeled fruits or vegetables (they may have been rinsed in contaminated water). Prophylactic drug therapy isn't recommended. Advise campers to purify all stream water before drinking it.

• Report epidemic situations to the public health authorities.

Toxoplasmosis

One of the most common infectious diseases, toxoplasmosis results from the protozoa *Toxoplasma gondii.* Distributed worldwide, it's less common in cold or hot, arid climates and at high elevations. It usually causes localized infection but may produce significant generalized infection, especially in immunodeficient patients or newborns. Congenital toxoplasmosis is characterized by lesions in the central nervous system and may result in stillbirth or serious birth defects.

Causes

T. gondii exists in trophozoite forms in the acute stages of infection and in cystic forms (tissue cysts and oocysts) in the latent stages. Ingestion of tissue cysts in raw or uncooked meat (heating, drying, or freezing destroys these cysts) or fecal-oral contamination from infected cats transmits toxoplasmosis. However, toxoplasmosis also occurs in vegetarians who aren't exposed to cats, so other means of transmission may exist. Congenital toxoplasmosis follows transplacental transmission from a chronically infected mother or one who acquired toxoplasmosis shortly before or during pregnancy.

Signs and symptoms

Toxoplasmosis acquired in the first trimester of pregnancy often results in stillbirth. About one-third of infants who survive have congenital toxoplasmosis. The later in pregnancy that maternal infection occurs, the greater the risk of congenital infection in the infant. Obvious signs of congenital toxoplasmosis include retinochoroiditis, hydrocephalus or microcephalus, cerebral calcification, seizures, lymphadenopathy, fever, hepatosplenomegaly, jaundice, and rash. Other defects, which may become apparent months or years later, include strabismus, blindness, epilepsy, and mental retardation. (See *Ocular toxoplasmosis*, page 184.)

Acquired toxoplasmosis may cause localized (mild lymphatic) or generalized (fulminating, disseminated) infection. Localized infection produces fever and a mononucleosis-like syndrome (malaise, myalgia, headache, fatigue, sore throat) and lymphadenopathy.

Generalized infection produces encephalitis, fever, headache, vomiting, delirium, seizures, and a diffuse maculopapular rash (except on the palms, soles, and scalp). Generalized infection may lead to myocarditis, pneumonitis, hepatitis, and polymyositis.

Diagnosis

Identification of *T. gondii* in an appropriate tissue specimen confirms toxoplasmosis. Serologic tests may be useful, and in patients with toxoplasmosis encephalitis, computed tomography and magnetic resonance imaging scans disclose lesions.

Treatment

Treatment for acute disease consists of drug therapy with sulfonamides and pyrimethamine for about 4 weeks and, possibly, folinic acid to control adverse effects. In patients who also have acquired immunodeficiency syndrome, treatment continues indefinitely. No safe, effective treatment exists for chronic toxoplasmosis or toxoplasmosis occurring in the first trimester of pregnancy.

Special considerations

• When caring for patients with toxoplasmosis, monitor drug therapy carefully and emphasize thorough patient teaching to prevent complications and control spread of the disease.
• Because sulfonamides cause blood dyscrasias and pyrimethamine depresses bone marrow, closely monitor the patient's hematologic values. Also emphasize the importance of regularly scheduled follow-up care.

Ocular toxoplasmosis

Characterized by focal necrotizing retinitis, ocular toxoplasmosis (active retinochoroiditis) accounts for about 25% of all granulomatous uveitis. It usually results from congenital infection, but may not appear until adolescence or young adulthood, when infection is reactivated.

Symptoms include blurred vision, scotoma, pain, photophobia, and impairment or loss of central vision. Vision improves as inflammation subsides but usually without recovery of lost visual acuity.

Ocular toxoplasmosis may subside after treatment with prednisone.

• Teach all persons to wash their hands after working with soil (because it may be contaminated with cat oocysts); to cook meat thoroughly and freeze it promptly if it's not for immediate use; to change cat litter daily (cat oocysts don't become infective until 1 to 4 days after excretion); to cover children's sandboxes; and to keep flies away from food (flies transport oocysts).

• Report all cases of toxoplasmosis to your local public health department.

Self-test questions

You can quickly review your comprehension of this chapter on protozoal infections by answering the following questions. The correct answers to these questions and their rationales appear on pages 227 to 230.

Case history questions

Tom Tucker, an HIV-infected adolescent, has developed Pneumocystis carinii pneumonia (PCP).

1. Tom is concerned about how he got PCP and states that he hasn't been around anyone with a cold recently. Which of the following explanations of transmission would you offer?
    a. He could have contracted it from a pet dog or cat.
    b. He was probably exposed to contaminated articles, such as drinking glasses or cups.
    c. The disease is readily transmitted from person to person among those who are immunosuppressed.

    d. The causative organism was probably already a normal resident in his lungs but caused disease because of his impaired immune system.

2. Early signs and symptoms of PCP include:
    a. increasing shortness of breath and a nonproductive cough.
    b. anorexia, generalized fatigue, and weight loss.
    c. high, remittent fever.
    d. hypoxemia with cyanosis and decreased breath sounds.

3. Tom's PCP could be confirmed by:
    a. chest X-ray.
    b. transbronchial biopsy.
    c. induced first-morning sputum specimen.
    d. gallium scanning.

4. Tom is initially treated with co-trimoxazole. To prevent bone marrow suppression, a severe reaction associated with this drug, he will also receive:
    a. leucovorin.
    b. folic acid.
    c. cyanocobalamin.
    d. pyridoxine.

5. Which drug was recently approved for alternative treatment of moderate to severe PCP?
    a. I.V. pentamidine.
    b. Aerosolized pentamidine.
    c. Vindesine sulfate.
    d. Trimetrexate glucuronate.

Additional questions

6. Unequivocal diagnosis of malaria depends on:
    a. a history of travel to endemic areas in a person with high fever of unknown origin.
    b. indirect fluorescent serum antibody tests.
    c. identification of the parasites in red blood cells.
    d. parasites in urine sediment.

7. Malaria is best treated with:
  a. oral quinine.
  b. oral chloroquine.
  c. I.M. chloroquine.
  d. primaquine.

8. *Entamoeba histolytica,* the causative agent in amebiasis, is spread by:
  a. airborne transmission.
  b. enteric transmission.
  c. contact transmission.
  d. vectorborne transmission.

9. In giardiasis, attachment of *G. lamblia* to the intestinal lumen causes superficial mucosal invasion and destruction, inflammation, and irritation resulting in:
  a. perforation.
  b. malabsorption.
  c. obstruction.
  d. hemorrhage.

10. During acute toxoplasmosis, treatment consists of drug therapy with:
  a. a 10-day course of metronidazole.
  b. emetine chloride in combination with tetracycline.
  c. iodoquinol.
  d. sulfonamides and pyrimethamine.

CHAPTER 6

Helminthic Infections

Infection with parasitic worms, such as the fluke, tapeworm, and roundworm, results in helminthic disorders.

Trichinosis

Also called trichiniasis and trichinellosis, trichinosis is caused by larvae of the intestinal roundworm *Trichinella spiralis*. It occurs worldwide, especially in populations that eat pork or bear meat. Trichinosis may produce multiple symptoms; respiratory, central nervous system (CNS), and cardiovascular complications; and, rarely, death.

Causes

Transmission results from ingestion of uncooked or undercooked meat that contains *T. spiralis* cysts. Such cysts are found primarily in swine, less often in dogs, cats, bears, foxes, wolves, and marine animals. These cysts result from the animals' ingestion of similarly contaminated flesh. In swine, such infection results from eating table scraps or raw garbage. After gastric juices free the worm from the cyst capsule, it reaches sexual maturity in a few days. The female roundworm burrows into the intestinal mucosa and reproduces. Larvae are then transported through the lymphatic system and the bloodstream. They become embedded as cysts in striated muscle, especially in the diaphragm, chest, arms, and legs. Human-to-human transmission does not take place.

Signs and symptoms

In the United States, trichinosis is usually mild and seldom produces symptoms. When symptoms do occur, they vary with the stage and degree of infection:

• Stage 1, invasion, occurs 1 week after ingestion. Release of larvae and reproduction of adult *T. spiralis* cause anorexia, nausea, vomiting, diarrhea, abdominal pain, and cramps.

• Stage 2, dissemination, occurs 7 to 10 days after ingestion. *T. spiralis* penetrates the intestinal mucosa and begins to migrate to striated muscle. Symptoms include edema, especially of the eyelids or face; muscle pain, particularly in the extremities; and, occasionally, itching and burning skin, sweating, skin lesions, a temperature of 102° to 104° F (38.8° to 40° C), and delirium; and, in severe respiratory, cardiovascular, or CNS infections, palpitations and lethargy.

• Stage 3, encystment, occurs during convalescence, generally 1 week later. *T. spiralis* larvae invade muscle fiber and become encysted.

Diagnosis

A history of ingestion of raw or improperly cooked pork or pork products, with typical clinical features, suggests trichinosis, but infection may be difficult to prove. Stools may contain mature worms and larvae during the invasion stage. Skeletal muscle biopsies can show encysted larvae 10 days after ingestion; and, if available, analyses of contaminated meat also show larvae.

Skin tests may show a positive histamine-like reactivity 15 minutes after intradermal injection of the antigen (within 17 to 20 days after ingestion). However, such a result may remain positive for up to 5 years after exposure. Elevated acute and convalescent antibody titers (determined by flocculation tests 3 to 4 weeks after infection) confirm this diagnosis.

Other abnormal results include elevated aspartate aminotransferase, alanine aminotransferase, creatine kinase, and lactate dehydrogenase levels during the acute stages and an elevated eosinophil count (up to 15,000/mm^3). A normal or increased cerebrospinal fluid lymphocyte level (to 300/mm^3) and increased protein levels indicate CNS involvement.

Treatment

Thiabendazole effectively combats this parasite during the intestinal stage; severe infection (especially CNS invasion) may warrant glucocorticoids to fight against possible inflammation.

**Special
considerations**

• Question the patient about recent ingestion of pork products and the methods used to store and cook them.
• Reduce fever with alcohol rubs, tepid baths, cooling blankets, or antipyretics; relieve muscular pain with analgesics, enforced bed rest, and proper body alignment.
• To prevent pressure ulcers, frequently reposition the patient, and gently massage bony prominences.
• Tell the patient that possible adverse effects of thiabendazole are nausea, vomiting, dizziness, dermatitis, and fever.
• Explain the importance of bed rest. Sudden death from cardiac involvement may occur in a patient with moderate to severe infection who has resumed activity too soon. Warn the patient to continue bed rest into the convalescent stage to avoid a serious relapse and possible death.
• To help prevent trichinosis, educate the public about proper cooking and storing methods not only for pork and pork products, but also for meat from carnivores. To kill trichinae, internal meat temperatures should reach 150° F (65.6° C) and its color should change from pink to grey unless the meat has been cured or frozen for at least 10 days at low temperatures.
• Warn travelers to foreign countries or to very poor areas in the United States to avoid eating pork; swine in these areas are often fed raw garbage.
• Report all cases of trichinosis to local public health authorities.

Hookworm disease

An infection of the upper intestine, hookworm disease (also called uncinariasis) is caused by *Ancylostoma duodenale* (found in the eastern hemisphere) or *Necator americanus* (in the western hemisphere). Sandy soil, high humidity, a warm climate, and failure to wear shoes all favor its transmission. In the United States, hookworm disease is most common in the southeast. Although this disease can cause cardiopulmonary complications, it's rarely fatal, except in debilitated persons or infants under age 1.

Causes

Both forms of hookworm disease are transmitted to humans through direct skin penetration (usually in the foot) by hookworm larvae in soil contaminated with feces containing hookworm ova. These ova develop into infectious larvae in 1 to 3 days.

Larvae travel through the lymphatic to the pulmonary capillaries, where they penetrate alveoli and move up the bronchial tree to the trachea and epiglottis. There they are swallowed and enter the GI tract. When they reach the small intestine, they mature, attach to the jejunal mucosa, and suck blood, oxygen, and glucose from the intestinal wall. These mature worms then deposit ova, which are excreted in the stool, starting the cycle anew. Hookworm larvae mature in approximately 5 to 6 weeks.

Signs and symptoms

Most cases of hookworm disease produce few symptoms and may be overlooked until worms are passed in stools. The earliest signs and symptoms include irritation, pruritus, and edema at the site of entry, which are sometimes accompanied by secondary bacterial infection with pustule formation.

When the larvae reach the lungs, they may cause pneumonitis and hemorrhage with fever, sore throat, crackles, and cough. Finally, intestinal infection may cause fatigue, nausea, weight loss, dizziness, melena, and uncontrolled diarrhea.

In severe and chronic infection, anemia from blood loss may lead to cardiomegaly (a result of increased oxygen demands), heart failure, and generalized massive edema.

Diagnosis

Identification of hookworm ova in stools confirms the diagnosis. Anemia suggests severe chronic infection. In infected patients, blood studies show:
• *hemoglobin* level of 5 to 9 g/dl (in severe cases)
• *leukocyte* count as high as 47,000/mm^3
• *eosinophil* count of 500 to 700/mm^3.

Treatment

Appropriate treatment for hookworm infection includes administering mebendazole or pyrantel and providing an iron-rich diet or iron supplements to prevent or correct anemia.

Special considerations

• Obtain a complete history, with special attention to travel or residency in endemic areas. Note the sequence and onset of symptoms. Interview the family and other close contacts to see if they too have any symptoms.

• Carefully examine the patient, noting signs of entry, lymphedema, and respiratory status.

• If the patient has confirmed hookworm infestation, segregate the incontinent patient.

• Wash your hands thoroughly after every patient contact.

• For severe anemia, administer oxygen, as needed, at low to moderate flow. Be sure the oxygen is humidified because the patient may already have upper airway irritation from the parasites.

• Encourage coughing and deep breathing to stimulate removal of blood or secretions from involved lung areas and to prevent secondary infection.

• Allow frequent rest periods because the patient may tire easily.

• If anemia causes immobility, reposition the patient often to prevent skin breakdown.

• Closely monitor intake and output. Note quantity and frequency of diarrheic stools. Dispose of feces promptly, and wear gloves when doing so.

• To help assess nutritional status, weigh the patient daily.

• To combat malnutrition, emphasize the importance of good nutrition, with particular attention to foods high in iron and protein.

• If the patient receives iron supplements, explain that they will darken stools.

• Administer anthelmintics on an empty stomach, but without a purgative.

• To help prevent reinfection, educate the patient in proper hand-washing technique and sanitary disposal of feces. Tell him to wear shoes in endemic areas.

Ascariasis

Also referred to as roundworm infection, ascariasis, an infection caused by *Ascaris lumbricoides*, occurs worldwide but is most common in tropical areas with poor sanitation and in Asia, where farmers use human feces as fertilizer. In the United States, it's more prevalent in the south, particularly among 5- to 12-year-olds.

Causes

A. lumbricoides is a large roundworm resembling an earthworm. It's transmitted to humans by ingestion of soil contaminated with human feces that harbor *A. lumbricoides* ova. Such ingestion may occur directly (by eating contaminated soil) or indirectly (by eating poorly washed raw vegetables grown in contaminated soil). Ascariasis never passes directly from person to person. After ingestion, *A. lumbricoides* ova hatch and release larvae, which penetrate the intestinal wall and reach the lungs through the bloodstream. After about 10 days in pulmonary capillaries and alveoli, the larvae migrate to the bronchioles, bronchi, trachea, and epiglottis. There they are swallowed and return to the intestine to mature into worms.

Signs and symptoms

Ascariasis produces two phases: early pulmonary and prolonged intestinal. Mild intestinal infection may cause only vague stomach discomfort. The first clue may be vomiting a worm or passing a worm in stools.

Severe infection, however, effects stomach pain, vomiting, restlessness, disturbed sleep, and, in extreme cases, intestinal obstruction. Larvae migrating by the lymphatic and the circulatory systems cause symptoms that vary; for instance, when they invade the lungs, pneumonitis may result.

Diagnosis

The key to diagnosis is identifying ova in stools or adult worms, which may be passed rectally or by mouth. When migrating larvae invade alveoli, other conclusive tests include X-rays that show characteristic bronchovascular markings: infiltrates, patchy areas of pneumonitis, and widening of hilar shadows. In a patient with ascariasis, these findings usually accompany a complete blood count that shows eosinophilia.

Treatment

Anti-*Ascaris* drug therapy, the primary treatment, uses pyrantel or piperazine to temporarily paralyze the worms, permitting peristalsis to expel them. Mebendazole is also used to block helminth nutrition. These drugs are up to 95% effective, even after a single dose. In multiple helminth infection, one of these drugs must be the first treatment; using some other anthelmintic first may stimulate *A. lumbricoides* perforation into other organs. No specific treatment exists for migratory infection, because anthelmintics affect only mature worms.

In intestinal obstruction, nasogastric (NG) suctioning controls vomiting. When suctioning can be discontinued, instill piperazine and clamp the tube. If vomiting does not occur, give a second dose of piperazine orally 24 hours later. If drug therapy is ineffective, treatment probably requires surgery.

Special considerations

• Although isolation is unnecessary, properly dispose of feces and soiled linen, and carefully wash your hands after patient contact.
• If the patient is receiving NG suctioning, be sure to give him good mouth care.
• Teach the patient to prevent reinfection by washing hands thoroughly, especially before eating and after defecation, and by bathing and changing underwear and bed linens daily.
• Inform the patient of the adverse effects of drugs. Tell him piperazine may cause stomach upset, dizziness, and urticaria. Remember, piperazine is contraindicated in convulsive disorders. Pyrantel produces red stools and vomit and may cause stomach upset, headache, dizziness, and skin rash; and mebendazole, abdominal pain and diarrhea.

Taeniasis

Also called tapeworm disease or cestodiasis, taeniasis is a parasitic infection by *Taenia saginata* (beef tapeworm), *T. solium* (pork tapeworm), *Diphyllobothrium latum* (fish tapeworm), or *Hymenolepis nana* (dwarf tapeworm). Taeniasis is usually a chronic, benign intestinal disease. *T. solium* may cause dangerous systemic and central nervous system (CNS) symptoms if larvae invade the brain and striated muscle of vital organs.

Causes

T. saginata, T. solium, and *D. latum* are transmitted to humans by ingestion of beef, pork, or fish that contains tapeworm cysts. Gastric acids break down these cysts in the stomach, liberating them to mature. Mature tapeworms fasten to the intestinal wall and produce ova that are passed in the feces. Transmission of *H. nana* is direct from person to person and requires no intermediate host; it completes its life cycle in the intestine. (See *Common tapeworm infestation.*)

Diagnosis

Tapeworm infestations require laboratory observation of tapeworm ova or body segments in feces for diagnosis. Because ova aren't excreted continuously, confirmation may require multiple specimens. A supporting dietary or travel history aids confirmation.

Treatment

In up to 95% of patients, treatment with niclosamide offers a cure. In beef, pork, and fish tapeworm infestation, the drug is given once; in severe dwarf tapeworm infestation, twice (5 to 7 days each time, spaced 2 weeks apart). Another anthelmintic agent, praziquantel, may also be effective.

During treatment for pork tapeworm, other health-related measures, such as laxative use or induced vomiting, are contraindicated because of the danger of autoinfection and systemic disease.

After drug treatment, all types of tapeworm infection require a follow-up laboratory examination of stool specimens during the next 3 to 5 weeks to check for any remaining ova or worm segments. Of course, persistent infection typically requires a second course of medication.

Common tapeworm infestation

TYPE	SOURCE OF INFECTION	INCIDENCE	CLINICAL FEATURES
Taenia saginata beef tapeworm	Uncooked or undercooked infected beef	Worldwide but prevalent in Europe and East Africa	Crawling sensation in the perianal area caused by worm segments that have been passed rectally; intestinal obstruction and appendicitis due to long worm segments that have twisted in the intestinal lumen
Taenia solium pork tapeworm	Uncooked or undercooked infected pork	Highest in Mexico, Latin America; lowest among Muslims and Jews	Seizures, headaches, personality changes; often overlooked in adults
Diphyllobothrium latum fish tapeworm	Uncooked or undercooked infected freshwater fish, such as pike, trout, salmon, and turbot	Finland, northern Russia, Japan, Alaska, Australia, the Great Lakes region (U.S.), Switzerland, Chile, and Argentina	Anemia (hemoglobin as low as 6 to 8 g)
Hymenolepis nana dwarf tapeworm	No intermediate host; parasite passes directly from person to person via ova passed in stools; inadequate hand washing facilitates its spread	Most common tapeworm in humans; particularly prevalent among institutionalized mentally retarded children and in underdeveloped countries	Dependent on patient's nutritional status and number of parasites; often no symptoms with mild infection; with severe infection, anorexia, diarrhea, restlessness, dizziness, and apathy

Special considerations

• Obtain a complete history, including recent travel to endemic areas, dietary habits, and physical symptoms.
• Dispose of the patient's excretions carefully. Wear gloves when giving personal care and handling fecal excretions, bedpans, and bed linens; wash your hands thoroughly and instruct the patient to do the same.
• Tell the patient not to consume anything after midnight on the day niclosamide therapy is to start, as the drug must be given on an empty stomach. After administering the drug, document passage of strobilae.

• In pork tapeworm infestation, use enteric and secretion precautions. Avoid procedures and drugs that may cause vomiting or gagging. If the patient is a child or is incontinent, he requires a private room. Obtain a list of contacts.

• Document level of consciousness, and report any changes immediately. If CNS symptoms appear, keep an artificial airway or padded tongue blade close at hand, raise side rails, keep the bed low, and help with walking as needed.

• To prevent reinfection, teach proper hand-washing technique and the need to cook meat and fish thoroughly.

• Stress the need for follow-up evaluations to monitor the success of therapy and to detect possible reinfection.

Enterobiasis

This benign intestinal disease is caused by the nematode *Enterobius vermicularis*. (Enterobiasis is also called pinworm, seatworm, or threadworm infection or oxyuriasis.) Found worldwide, it's common even in temperate regions with good sanitation. It's the most prevalent helminthic infection in the United States.

Causes

Adult pinworms live in the intestine; female worms migrate to the perianal region to deposit their ova. Direct transmission occurs when the patient's hands transfer infective eggs from the anus to the mouth. Indirect transmission occurs when he comes in contact with contaminated articles, such as linens and clothing. Enterobiasis infection and reinfection occurs most often in children between ages 5 and 14 and in certain institutionalized groups because of poor hygiene and frequent hand-to-mouth activity. Crowded living conditions often enhance its spread to several members of a family.

Signs and symptoms

Asymptomatic enterobiasis is often overlooked. However, intense perianal pruritus may occur, especially at night, when the female worm crawls out of the anus to deposit ova. Pruritus disturbs sleep and causes irritability, scratching, skin irritation, and sometimes, vaginitis. Rarely, complications include appendicitis, salpingitis, and pelvic granuloma.

Diagnosis

A history of pruritus ani suggests enterobiasis; identification of *Enterobius* ova recovered from the perianal area with a cellophane tape swab confirms it. In this test, cellophane tape is placed sticky-side out on the base end of a test tube, and the tube is rolled around the perianal region. The tape is then examined under a microscope. This test should be done before the patient bathes and defecates in the morning. A stool sample is generally ova and worm free, because these worms deposit the ova outside the intestine and die after migration to the anus.

Treatment

Drug therapy with pyrantel, piperazine, or mebendazole destroys these parasites. Effective eradication requires simultaneous treatment of family members and, in institutions, other patients.

Special considerations

• If the patient receives pyrantel, tell him and his family that this drug colors stools bright red and may cause vomiting (vomitus will also be red). The tablet form of this drug is coated with aspirin and shouldn't be given to aspirin-sensitive patients.

• Before giving piperazine, obtain a history of convulsive disorders. Piperazine may aggravate these disorders and is contraindicated in a patient with such a history.

• To help prevent this disease, tell parents to bathe children daily (showers are preferable to tub baths) and to change underwear and bed linens daily.

• Educate children in proper personal hygiene, and stress the need for hand washing after defecation and before handling food.

• Discourage nail biting. If the child can't stop, suggest that he wear gloves until the infection clears.

• Report *all* outbreaks of enterobiasis to school authorities.

Schistosomiasis

A slowly progressive disease, Schistosomiasis (bilharziasis) is caused by blood flukes of the class *Trematoda*. These parasites are of three major types: *Schistosoma mansoni* and *S. japonicum* infect the intestinal tract; *S. haematobium* infects the urinary tract. The degree of infection determines the intensity of illness. Complications — such as portal hypertension, pulmonary hypertension, heart failure, ascites, hematemesis from ruptured esophageal varies, and renal failure — can be fatal.

Causes

The mode of transmission is bathing, swimming, wading, or working in water contaminated with *Schistosoma* larvae, known (while infective) as cercariae. These cercariae penetrate the skin or mucous membranes and eventually work their way to the liver's venous portal circulation. There, they mature in 1 to 3 months. The adults then migrate to other parts of the body.

The female cercariae lay spiny eggs in blood vessels surrounding the large intestine or bladder. After penetrating the mucosa of these organs, the eggs are excreted in feces or urine. If the eggs hatch in fresh water, the first-stage larvae (miracidia) penetrate freshwater snails, which act as passive intermediate hosts. Cercariae produced in snails escape into water and begin a new life cycle. (See *Types of schistosomes.*)

Signs and symptoms

Clinical features of schistosomiasis depend on the site of infection and the stage of the disease. Initially, a transient, pruritic rash develops at the site of cercariae penetration, along with fever, myalgia, and cough. Worm migration and egg deposition may cause such complications as flaccid paralysis, seizures, and skin abscesses. (See *Schistosomal dermatitis*, page 200.)

Diagnosis

Typical symptoms and a history of travel to endemic areas suggest the diagnosis; ova in the urine or stool or a mucosal lesion biopsy confirms it. A white blood cell count shows eosinophilia.

Types of schistosomes

SPECIES AND INCIDENCE	SIGNS AND SYMPTONS	TREATMENT	ADVERSE EFFECTS
Schistosoma mansoni Western hemisphere, particularly Puerto Rico, Lesser Antilles, Brazil, and Venezuela; also the Nile Delta, Sudan, and central Africa	Irregular fever, malaise, weakness, abdominal distress, weight loss, diarrhea, ascites, hepatosplenomegaly, portal hypertension, fistulae, intestinal stricture	Praziquantel; oxamniquine P.O.	Headache, abdominal pain, drowsiness, nausea, vomiting, anorexia, weakness, diarrhea, lassitude, myalgia
S. japonicum Affects men more than women; particularly prevalent among farmers in Japan, China, and the Philippines	Irregular fever, malaise, weakness, abdominal distress, weight loss, diarrhea, ascites, hepatosplenomegaly, portal hypertension, fistulae, intestinal stricture	Praziquantel; niridazole P.O.; stibocaptate (rare)	Headache, abdominal pain, drowsiness, nausea, thrombocytopenia, hypotension, syncope, bradycardia, ECG changes, vomiting, diarrhea, colic, hepatic necrosis, dyspnea, severe arthralgia, albuminuria, fever, dermatitis
S. haematobium Africa, Cyprus, Greece, India	Terminal hematuria, dysuria, ureteral colic; with secondary infection—colicky pain, intermittent flank pain, vague GI complaints, total renal failure	Praziquantel; metrifonate P.O.; niridazole P.O.	Headache, abdominal pain, drowsiness, nausea, vomiting, diarrhea, anorexia, dizziness, insomnia, cardiac arrhythmia, anxiety, confusion, hallucinations, seizures

Treatment

The treatment of choice is the anthelmintic drug praziquantel. Three to six months after treatment, the patient will need to be examined again. If this checkup detects any living eggs, treatment may be resumed.

Special considerations

• To help prevent schistosomiasis, teach those in endemic areas to work for a pure water supply and to avoid contaminated water. If they must enter this water, tell them to wear protective clothing and to dry themselves afterward.

Schistosomal dermatitis

This form of dermatitis, also known as swimmer's itch or clam digger's itch, affects those who bathe in and camp along freshwater lakes in the eastern and western United States.

It's caused by a schistosomal cercaria that is harbored by migratory birds and can penetrate the skin, causing a pruritic papular rash. Initially mild, the reaction grows more severe with repeated exposure.

Treatment consists of 5% copper sulfate solution as an antipruritic and 2% methylene blue as an antibacterial agent.

Strongyloidiasis

Also called threadworm infection, strongyloidiasis is a parasitic intestinal infection caused by the helminth *Strongyloides stercoralis*. This worldwide infection is endemic in the tropics and subtropics. Susceptibility to strongyloidiasis is universal. Infection doesn't confer immunity, and immunocompromised persons may suffer overwhelming disseminated infection. Because the threadworm's reproductive cycle may continue in the untreated host for up to 45 years, autoinfection is highly probable. Most patients with strongyloidiasis recover, but debilitation from protein loss may result in death.

Causes

Transmission to humans usually occurs through contact with soil that contains infective *S. stercoralis* filariform larvae; such larvae develop from noninfective rhabdoid (rod-shaped) larvae in human feces. The filariform larvae penetrate the human skin, usually at the feet, then migrate by way of the lymphatic system to the bloodstream and the lungs.

Once they enter into pulmonary circulation, the filariform larvae break through the alveoli and migrate upward to the pharynx, where they are swallowed. Then, they lodge in the small intestine, where they deposit eggs that mature into noninfectious rhabdoid larvae. Next, these larvae migrate into the large intestine and are excreted in feces, starting the cycle again. The threadworm life cycle—which begins with penetration of the skin and ends with excretion of rhabdoid larvae—takes 17 days.

In autoinfection, rhabdoid larvae mature within the intestine to become infective filariform larvae.

Signs and symptoms

The patient's resistance and the extent of infection determine the severity of symptoms. Some patients have no symptoms, but many develop an erythematous maculopapular rash at the site of penetration that produces swelling and pruritus and that may be confused with an insect bite. As the larvae migrate to the lungs, pulmonary signs develop, including minor hemorrhage, pneumonitis, and pneumonia; later, intestinal infection produces frequent, watery, and bloody diarrhea, accompanied by intermittent abdominal pain.

Severe infection can cause malnutrition from substantial fat and protein loss, anemia, and lesions resembling ulcerative colitis, all of which invite secondary bacterial infection. Ulcerated intestinal mucosa may lead to perforation and, possibly, potentially fatal dissemination, especially in patients with malignancy or immunodeficiency diseases or in those who receive immunosuppressants.

Diagnosis

In strongyloidiasis, diagnosis requires observation of *S. stercoralis* larvae in a fresh stool specimen (2 hours after excretion, rhabdoid larvae look like hookworm larvae). During the pulmonary phase, sputum may show many eosinophils and larvae; marked eosinophilia also occurs in disseminated strongyloidiasis.

Other helpful tests include:
• *chest X-ray* (positive during pulmonary phase of infection)
• *hemoglobin level* (as low as 6 to 10 g/dl)
• *white blood cell count with differential* (eosinophils 450 to 700/mm^3).

Treatment

Because of potential autoinfection, treatment with thiabendazole is required for 2 to 3 days (total dose not to exceed 3 g). Patients also need protein replacement, blood transfusions, and I.V. fluids. Retreatment is necessary if *S. stercoralis* remains in stools after therapy. Glucocorticoids are contraindicated because they increase the risk of autoinfection and dissemination.

Special
considerations

• Keep accurate intake and output records.
• The patient will need a high protein diet and, to increase caloric intake, perhaps tube feedings.
• Wear gloves when giving perineal care.
• Because direct person-to-person transmission doesn't occur, isolation is not required.
• Label stool specimens for laboratory as contaminated.
• Warn the patient that thiabendazole may cause mild nausea, vomiting, drowsiness, and giddiness.
• In pulmonary infection, reposition the patient frequently, and encourage coughing and deep breathing.
• To prevent reinfection, teach the patient proper handwashing technique. Stress the importance of washing hands before eating and after defecating, and of wearing shoes when in endemic areas.
• Check the patient's family for signs of infection.
• Follow-up stool examination is necessary for several weeks after treatment.

Self-test questions

You can quickly review your comprehension of this chapter on helminthic infections by answering the following questions. The correct answers to these questions and their rationales appear on pages 230 to 233.

Case history
questions

James Brown, age 56, comes to the outpatient department complaining of loss of appetite, nausea, vomiting, diarrhea, abdominal pain, and cramps. He frequently eats pork and pork products and has been cooking for himself since his wife died 2 weeks ago. Trichinosis is suspected.

1. Mr. Brown's symptoms relate to which stage of trichinosis infection?
    a. Stage 1
    b. Stage 2
    c. Stage 3
    d. Stage 4

2. What frees the *Trichinella spiralis* roundworm from its cyst capsule?
  a. Heating the meat
  b. Salivary juices during chewing
  c. Gastric juices
  d. Duodenal and jejunal secretions

3. Trichinae larvae are transported:
  a. person-to-person.
  b. through the GI tract.
  c. through the lymphatic system and bloodstream.
  d. via animals ingesting contaminated raw garbage or table scraps.

4. Mr. Brown will benefit from treatment with:
  a. glucocorticoids.
  b. thiabendazole.
  c. mebendazole.
  d. piperazine.

Billy Boyd, age 9, is brought to your outpatient facility by his mother because she noted worms, and possibly their eggs, and what she thought might be blood in his stools. The boy denies any symptoms, but his mother says he seems tired, and you note that his skin and mucous membranes appear quite pale. Hookworm disease is suspected.

5. As an important part of history taking, you will ask Billy:
  a. "What kind of meat do you eat?"
  b. "Do you ever eat unwashed raw vegetables?"
  c. "Do you sleep with your brother or share clothing with him?"
  d. "Have you been walking barefoot outdoors?"

6. Hookworm larvae enter the GI tract to mature and deposit their ova by:
  a. traveling through blood and lymphatic channels.
  b. being swallowed after moving up the bronchial tree.
  c. direct hand transmission from anus to mouth.
  d. migrating from the liver's portal circulation.

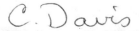

7. In addition to mebendazole or pyrantel to treat his hookworm infection, Billy will need:
   a. an iron-rich diet or iron supplements to prevent or correct anemia.
   b. alcohol rubs or tepid baths and antipyretics to reduce fever.
   c. nasogastric suction to control vomiting if he develops intestinal obstruction.
   d. to avoid laxatives or induced vomiting because of the danger of autoinfection.

Additional
questions

8. Before treating tapeworm disease with niclosamide, you will tell the patient to:
   a. drink at least 2 quarts (2 liters) of water after taking the drug to prevent renal crystallization.
   b. refrain from eating and drinking after midnight on the day that therapy is to begin because the drug must be taken on an empty stomach.
   c. obtain a follow-up examination in 3 to 6 months. It may be necessary to resume treatment if living eggs are found.
   d. follow a high protein diet for the duration of treatment. He may also require blood transfusion and I.V. fluids.

9. Before piperazine is prescribed, you must determine if the patient has a history of:
   a. hearing problems.
   b. hypertension.
   c. seizure disorders.
   d. coagulopathy.

10. Diagnosis of strongyloidosis (threadworm infection) requires:
   a. identification of ova in the urine or stools.
   b. recovery of ova from the perianal area with a cellophane tape swab.
   c. laboratory observation of ova or worm body segments in feces.
   d. a fresh stool specimen.

CHAPTER 7

Miscellaneous Infections

This category includes ornithosis, toxic shock syndrome, and Rocky Mountain spotted fever.

Ornithosis

Caused by the gram-negative intracellular parasite *Chlamydia psittaci*, ornithosis (also called psittacosis and parrot fever) is transmitted by infected birds. This disease occurs worldwide and is mainly associated with occupational exposure to birds (such as poultry farming). Incidence is higher in women and in persons ages 20 to 50. With adequate antimicrobial therapy, ornithosis is fatal in less than 4% of patients.

Causes

Psittacine birds (parrots, parakeets, cockatoos), pigeons, and turkeys may harbor *C. psittaci* in their blood, feathers, tissues, nasal secretions, liver, spleen, and feces. Transmission to humans occurs primarily through inhalation of dust containing *C. psittaci* from bird droppings and, less often, through direct contact with infected secretions or body tissues, as in laboratory personnel who work with birds. Rarely, person-to-person transmission occurs, usually causing severe ornithosis.

Signs and symptoms

After an incubation period of 4 to 15 days, onset of symptoms may be insidious or sudden. Clinical effects include chills and a low-grade fever that increases to 103° to 105° F (39.4° to 40.5° C) for 7 to 10 days, and then, with treatment, declines during the second or third week.

Other signs include headache, myalgia, sore throat, cough (may be dry, hacking, and nonproductive, or may produce blood-tinged sputum), abdominal distention and tenderness, nausea, vomiting, photophobia, decreased pulse rate, slightly increased respirations, secondary purulent lung infection, and a faint macular rash.

Severe infection also produces delirium, stupor, and, in extensive pulmonary infiltration, cyanosis. Ornithosis may recur, but is usually milder.

Diagnosis

The above symptoms and a recent history of exposure to birds suggest ornithosis.

Firm diagnosis requires recovery of *C. psittaci* from mice, eggs, or tissue culture inoculated with the patient's blood or sputum. Comparison of acute and convalescent serum shows a fourfold rise in *Chlamydia* antibody titers. In addition, a patchy lobar infiltrate appears on chest X-rays during the first week of illness.

Treatment

Ornithosis calls for treatment with tetracycline. If the infection is severe, tetracycline may be given I.V. until the fever subsides. Fever and other symptoms should begin to subside 48 to 72 hours after antibiotic treatment begins; but treatment must continue for 2 weeks after temperature returns to normal. If the patient can't tolerate tetracycline, penicillin G procaine or chloramphenicol is an alternative.

Special considerations

• Monitor fluid and electrolyte balance. Give I.V. fluids as needed.

• Carefully monitor vital signs. Watch for signs of overwhelming infection.

• Reduce fever with tepid alcohol or sponge baths and a cooling blanket.

• Reposition the patient often.

• Observe secretion precautions. During the acute, febrile stage, if the patient has a cough, wear a face mask and wash your hands carefully. Instruct him to use tissues when he coughs and to dispose of them in a closed plastic bag.

• To prevent ornithosis, those who raise birds for sale should feed them tetracycline-treated birdseed and follow regulations on bird importation. They should segregate infected or

possibly infected birds from healthy birds, and disinfect structures that housed infected ones.
• Report all cases of ornithosis.

Toxic shock syndrome

An acute bacterial infection, toxic shock syndrome (TSS) is caused by toxin-producing, penicillin-resistant strains of *Staphylococcus aureus,* such as TSS toxin-1 and staphylococcal enterotoxins B and C. The disease primarily affects menstruating women under age 30 and is associated with continuous use of tampons during the menstrual period. TSS incidence peaked in the mid-1980s and has since declined, probably because of the withdrawal of high-absorbency tampons from the market.

Causes

Although tampons are clearly implicated in TSS, their exact role is uncertain. Theoretically, tampons may contribute to development of TSS by:
• introducing *S. aureus* into the vagina during insertion.
• absorbing toxin from the vagina.
• traumatizing the vaginal mucosa during insertion, thus leading to infection.
• providing a favorable environment for the growth of *S. aureus.*

When TSS isn't related to menstruation, it seems to be linked to *S. aureus* infections, such as abscesses, osteomyelitis, and postsurgical infections.

Signs and symptoms

Typically, TSS produces intense myalgias, fever over 104° F (40° C), vomiting, diarrhea, headache, decreased level of consciousness, rigors, conjunctival hyperemia, and vaginal hyperemia and discharge. Severe hypotension occurs with hypovolemic shock. Within a few hours of onset, a deep red rash develops — especially on the palms and soles — and later desquamates.

Major complications include persistent neuropsychological abnormalities, mild renal failure, rash, and cyanotic arms and legs.

Diagnosis

Firm diagnosis will center on clinical findings and the presence of at least three of the following:
• GI effects, including vomiting and profuse diarrhea
• muscular effects, with severe myalgias or a fivefold or greater increase in creatine kinase level
• mucous membrane effects, such as frank hyperemia
• renal involvement with elevated blood urea nitrogen or creatinine levels (at least thrice the normal levels)
• liver involvement with elevated bilirubin, aspartate aminotransferase or alanine aminotransferase levels (at least twice the normal levels)
• blood involvement with signs of thrombocytopenia and a platelet count of less than 100,000/mm³
• central nervous system effects, such as disorientation without focal signs.

In addition, isolation of *S. aureus* from vaginal discharge or lesions helps support the diagnosis. Negative results on blood tests for Rocky Mountain spotted fever, leptospirosis, and measles help rule out these disorders.

Treatment

In TSS, treatment consists of I.V. antistaphylococcal antibiotics that are beta-lactamase–resistant, such as oxacillin and nafcillin. To reverse shock, expect to replace fluids with saline solution and colloids.

Special considerations

• Monitor the patient's vital signs frequently.
• Administer antibiotics slowly and strictly on time. Be sure to watch for signs of penicillin allergy.
• Check the patient's fluid and electrolyte balance.
• Obtain specimens of vaginal and cervical secretions for culture of *S. aureus.*
• Tell the patient to avoid tampons.
• Implement universal precautions.

Rocky Mountain spotted fever

This febrile, rash-producing illness is caused by *Rickettsia rickettsii*. Rocky Mountain spotted fever (RMSF) is transmitted to humans by a tick bite. Endemic throughout the continental United States, RMSF is particularly prevalent in the southeast and southwest. RMSF is associated with outdoor activities, such as camping, backpacking, and hiking. Because of this, the incidence of this illness is usually higher in the spring and summer months. Epidemiologic surveillance reports for RMSF indicate that the incidence is also higher in children ages 5 to 9, men and boys, and whites. (See *Rocky Mountain spotted fever: Tracing its rise and fall,* page 210.)

RMSF is fatal in about 5% of patients. Mortality rises when treatment is delayed; it also increases in older patients.

Causes

R. rickettsii is transmitted by the wood tick (*Dermacentor andersoni*) in the west and by the dog tick (*D. variabilis*) in the east. RMSF is transmitted to a human or small animal by a prolonged bite (4 to 6 hours) of an adult tick.

Occasionally, RMSF is acquired through inhalation or through contact of abraded skin with tick excreta or tissue juices. (This explains why people shouldn't crush ticks between their fingers when removing them from other people and animals.) In most tick-infested areas, 1% to 5% of the ticks harbor *R. rickettsii*.

Signs and symptoms

The incubation period is usually about 7 days, but it can range anywhere from 2 to 14 days. Generally, the shorter the incubation time, the more severe the infection. Symptoms usually begin abruptly and include a persistent fever of 102° to 104° F (38.8° to 40° C); a generalized, excruciating headache; and aching in the bones, muscles, joints, and back. In addition to these symptoms, the tongue is covered with a thick white coating that gradually turns brown as the fever persists and rises.

Initially, the skin may simply appear flushed. But between days 2 and 5, eruptions begin around the wrists, ankles, or forehead and, within 2 days, cover the entire body, including the scalp, palms, and soles. The rash consists of

Rocky Mountain spotted fever: Tracing its rise and fall

According to the Centers for Disease Control and Prevention, reported cases of Rocky Mountain spotted fever are either cyclical or declining—probably as a result of public health education efforts. The graph below plots the fever's incidence (per population of 10,000) in the United States over 70 years.

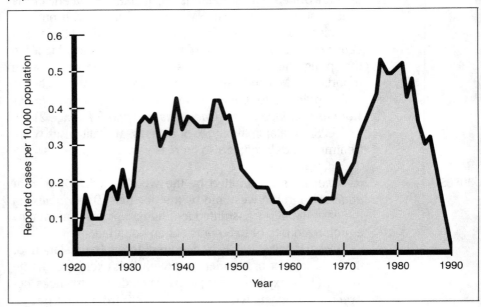

erythematous macules 1 to 5 mm in diameter that blanch on pressure; if untreated, the rash may become petechial and maculopapular. By the third week, the rash will cause the skin to peel off. Skin may become gangrenous over the elbows, fingers, and toes.

The pulse is strong initially, but it gradually becomes rapid (possibly reaching a rate of 150 beats/minute) and thready. A rapid pulse rate and hypotension (less than 90 mm Hg systolic) herald imminent death resulting from vascular collapse.

Other signs and symptoms include a bronchial cough, a rapid respiratory rate (as high as 60 breaths/minute), anorexia, nausea, vomiting, constipation, abdominal pain, hepatomegaly, splenomegaly, insomnia, restlessness and, in extreme cases, delirium. Urine output falls to half of the normal level or less, and the urine is dark and contains albumin.

Complications, although uncommon, include lobar pneumonia, otitis media, parotitis, disseminated intravascular coagulation (DIC), and possibly renal failure. In rare cases, RMSF leads to death.

Diagnosis

A positive diagnosis of RMSF generally rests on a history of a tick bite or travel to a tick-infested area. Also, a positive complement fixation test (which shows a fourfold increase in convalescent antibody titer compared with acute titers) should be obtained. Blood cultures should be performed to isolate the organism and confirm the diagnosis.

Another common but less reliable antibody test is the Weil-Felix reaction, which also shows a fourfold increase between the acute and convalescent sera titer levels. Increased titers usually develop after 10 to 14 days and persist for several months.

Additional recommended laboratory tests consist of a platelet count for thrombocytopenia (12,000 to 150,000/mm^3) and a white blood cell count (elevated to 11,000 to 33,000/mm^3). These two tests should be performed during the second week of illness.

Treatment

Appropriate treatment requires careful removal of the tick and administration of antibiotics, such as chloramphenicol or tetracycline, until 3 days after the fever subsides. Treatment also includes symptomatic measures and, in DIC, heparin and platelet transfusion.

Special considerations

• Carefully monitor the patient's intake and output. Watch closely for decreased urine output—a possible indicator of renal failure.

• Be alert for signs of dehydration, such as poor skin turgor and dry mouth.

• Administer antipyretics and provide tepid sponge baths to reduce fever.

• Monitor vital signs, and watch for profound hypotension and shock.

• Be prepared to administer oxygen therapy and assisted ventilation if pulmonary complications should develop.

• Turn the patient frequently to help prevent such possible complications of immobility as pressure ulcers and pneumonia.

• Pay close attention to the patient's nutritional needs because vomiting may necessitate I.V. nutrition or frequent small meals.

• Provide meticulous mouth care and other oral hygiene measures.

• When the patient recovers sufficiently, initiate disease-prevention and patient-teaching measures.

• If symptoms recur, instruct the patient to report them immediately. It's essential that treatment measures resume promptly.

• Advise the patient to avoid tick-infested areas if possible. Such areas may include woods, meadows, streams, and canyons.

• If the patient can't avoid tick-infested areas, make sure he knows how to protect himself from a prolonged tick bite, as follows:

— Encourage him to inspect his entire body (including his scalp) every 3 to 4 hours for attached ticks.

— Remind him to wear protective clothing, covering as much of his body as possible. He should wear a long-sleeved shirt, slacks securely tucked into laced boots, and a protective head covering, such as a hat, cap, or bandana.

— Advise him to apply insect repellant to exposed skin and even to his clothing.

— Tell him to receive vaccination (if available) against RMSF if he is planning an extended camping trip and will be far from adequate medical facilities.

• Offer printed and illustrated instructions, if available, that teach the patient and his family members or other caregivers how to correctly and safely remove a tick. Or show them how to use tweezers or forceps and how to apply steady traction to release the whole tick without leaving its mouth parts still in the skin.

• After the patient removes the tick, caution him not to handle it or its fragments.

• Finally, instruct the patient to clean his skin with alcohol at the point of attachment.

Self-test questions

You can quickly review your comprehension of this chapter on miscellaneous infections by answering the following questions. The correct answers to these questions and their rationales appear on pages 233 and 234.

Case history questions

Carl and Sylvia Mosner, ages 48 and 51, both became ill with headache, sore throat, cough, muscle aches, chills, and increasing fever. About 2 weeks earlier, they'd received a parrot as a gift from a friend who is a sea captain. After hearing their symptoms, their doctor suspected parrot fever.

1. Ornithosis, caused by the gram-negative intracellular parasite *Chlamydia psittaci,* is transmitted from infected birds to humans primarily through:
  a. person-to-person contact.
  b. direct contact with infected secretions or body tissues.
  c. occupational exposure to birds (poultry farmers, for example).
  d. inhalation of contaminated dust from bird droppings.

2. What other signs and symptoms would you expect to find?
  a. Abdominal distention and tenderness
  b. Diarrhea
  c. Tachycardia and bradypnea
  d. Vesicular rash

3. A confirming diagnosis of parrot fever requires recovery of *C. psittaci* from:
  a. bird droppings.
  b. tissue culture inoculated with the patient's blood or sputum.
  c. mice or eggs inoculated with bird blood or sputum.
  d. bird liver cells showing microscopic evidence of the intracellular parasite.

4. The most effective treatment for ornithosis is drug therapy with oral or I.V.:
  a. penicillin G.
  b. chloramphenicol.
  c. methicillin.
  d. tetracycline.

Ann Quigley, age 23, developed intense muscle aches, headache, fever, vomiting, and diarrhea this morning. Feeling dizzy and confused, Ann asked her roommate to drive her to the emergency unit. On arrival at your facility, Ann's temperature is 104° F (40° C); her pulse, 128 and thready; and her respirations, 28. Her blood pressure is 70/50 mm Hg. Ann's roommate says that number sounds low, that Ann's blood pressure is usually "90 over something."

5. In taking a history, you will try to determine:
  a. whether she has been exposed to anyone with similar symptoms.
  b. if she is menstruating and whether or not she uses tampons.
  c. her immunization history, especially for rubeola and rubella.
  d. whether she has been traveling outside of the continental United States.

6. Which of the following symptoms would you assess for in your physical examination?
  a. Conjunctival pallor
  b. Vaginal hyperemia
  c. Nuchal rigidity
  d. Anuria

7. As you initiate fluid replacement therapy for Ann, you note the onset of a rash that is typical of toxic shock syndrome (TSS). It appears:
  a. vesicular and located on the oropharynx and labia.
  b. macular, starting on the patient's face and then generalizing.
  c. deep red in color and located primarily on her palms and soles.

d. localized as vesicular lesions, confined to one dermatome.

8. After taking a vaginal culture to isolate *S. aureus* to confirm the TSS diagnosis, you initiate treatment with a beta-lactamase-resistant antibiotic such as:
   a. ampicillin or amoxicillin.
   b. methicillin or dicloxacillin.
   c. oxacillin or nafcillin.
   d. carbenicillin or mezlocillin.

While on a weekend hiking trip with his family, 7-year-old Alex Cunningham is bitten by a wood tick. Several days later, Alex develops a fever of 102° F (38.9° C), an excruciating headache, and aches and pains. In addition, his tongue becomes covered with a thick white coating and erythematous macules appear on his wrists, ankles, and forehead. Concerned about his symptoms, Mrs. Cunningham takes her son to see the pediatrician. Noting the history of a recent tick bite and current symptoms, along with the physical findings of tongue coating and erythematous macules, the doctor suspects the child has Rocky Mountain spotted fever and orders blood cultures to confirm the diagnosis of this disorder.

9. Which of the following statements accurately describes this rickettsia infection?
   a. Rocky Mountain spotted fever can also be transmitted through the bite of a deer tick.
   b. Generally, the shorter the incubation time, the milder the infection.
   c. Although uncommon, disseminated intravascular coagulation may occur as a result of Rocky Mountain spotted fever.
   d. Rocky Mountain spotted fever is transmitted to a human by the bite of an adult tick that lasts less than 5 seconds.

10. Which of the following antibiotics are commonly used to treat Rocky Mountain spotted fever?
   a. Tetracycline
   b. Erythromycin
   c. Amantadine
   d. Amphotericin B

Selected References
and Self-Test Answers and Rationales

Selected References

Balazs, A. "CMV Myocarditis in a Patient with HIV Disease," *AIDS Patient Care* 7(6):302-03, December 1993.

Bartlet, J. *Pocketbook of Infectious Disease Therapy.* Baltimore: Williams & Wilkins Co., 1994.

Duchin, J.S., et al. "Hantavirus Pulmonary Syndrome: A Clinical Description of 17 Patients with a Newly Recognized Disease," *New England Journal of Medicine* 330(14):949-55, April 7, 1994.

Fink, M.P. "Immunotherapy of Septic Shock," *Current Opinion in Anaesthesiology* 6(2):315-23, April 1993.

Gorbach, S.L., et al., eds. *Infectious Diseases.* Philadelphia: W.B. Saunders Co., 1992.

"Hantavirus Pulmonary Syndrome—United States, 1993," *MMWR* 43(3):45-48, January 28, 1994.

"Infection: An Old Problem Stages a Comeback," *Mayo Clinic Health Letter* 12(2):1-3, February 1994.

Isselbacher, K., et al., eds. *Harrison's Principles of Internal Medicine,* 13th ed. New York: McGraw-Hill Book Co., 1994.

Mandell, G.L., et al., eds. *Principles and Practice of Infectious Diseases: Antimicrobial Therapy 1993/1994.* New York: Churchill Livingstone, 1993.

Mocsny, N. "Nursing Considerations in the Treatment of Pneumocystis Carinii Pneumonia," *AIDS Patient Care* 7(5):259-61, October 1993.

Shulman, S.T., et al., eds. *The Biologic and Clinical Basis of Infectious Diseases,* 4th ed. Philadelphia: W.B. Saunders Co., 1992.

Smith, T.F., et al. "New Developments in the Diagnosis of Viral Diseases," *Infectious Disease Clinics of North America* 7(2):183-201, June 1993.

Stenberg, M.J. "Postoperative Pneumonia," *Today's OR Nurse* 15(5):19-22, September-October 1993.

Tanabe, P. "Commentary on Patient Assessment: Infection in the Elderly" [original article by Fraser, D. appears in *Journal of Gerontological Nursing 1993* 19(7):5-11, 44-45] *ENA's Nursing Scan in Emergency Care* 3(6):21, November-December 1993.

Self-Test Answers and Rationales

Chapter 1: Introduction

1. c The severity of an infection depends on three factors: the pathogenicity (ability to produce disease or virulence), number of invading microorganisms, and the strength of the host's defenses or resistance. This is sometimes expressed by the formula: $D = NV/R$. Although infection still accounts for much serious illness, even in industrialized nations, it is a critical health care problem in developing countries. Invasion of the body by microorganisms that subsequently multiply without immune response indicates colonization. To be considered an infection, microorganisms must produce signs and symptoms as well as an immunologic response. One reason that disease-causing microorganisms are difficult to overcome is that some (but not most) bacteria develop resistance to antibiotics.

2. d An endogenous infection results when the host's naturally occurring flora is displaced from its usual site (such as when *E. coli* is displaced from the colon to the urinary tract). An exogenous infection is caused by environmental pathogens. A subclinical infection is one that has been verified by laboratory methods, although it causes no symptoms (described as "silent," or asymptomatic). A latent infection occurs after the causative microorganisms have lain dormant in the host, sometimes for many years.

3. d Although protozoa are the simplest single-cell organisms of the animal kingdom, they show a high level of cellular specialization. Like other animal cells, they have cell membranes rather than cell walls, and their nuclei are surrounded by nuclear membranes. Bacteria are single-cell microorganisms with well-defined cell walls. Chlamydiae are smaller than both bacteria and rickettsiae but larger than viruses. They, like viruses, depend on hosts for replication; unlike viruses, however, they are susceptible to antibiotics. Fungi are also single-cell organisms, whose nuclei are enveloped by nuclear membranes. They have rigid cell walls (as do plant cells), but they lack chlorophyll and show little cellular specialization.

4. d Vectorborne transmission refers to the transfer of disease organisms by an intermediate carrier (a vector), such as a flea or a mosquito. Transmission of infectious diseases via contaminated inanimate objects is called indirect contact, which is actually a form of contact transmission. Airborne transmission results from inhalation of contaminated aerosolized droplets. Oral-fecal (enteric) transmission occurs when organisms normally found in feces are ingested by susceptible individuals through contaminated food or water.

5. a Nosocomial infections, those acquired in a hospital or other health care facility, are usually transmitted by direct contact. Less often, transmission occurs by inhalation or indirect contact with contaminated equipment. Although *E. coli,* gram-negative colonic bacteria, are frequently determined to cause nosocomial infection, the primary mode of transmission for this organism in institutions is by direct or indirect contact, rather than by enteric transmission.

6. b In suspected infection, take the patient's temperature using the same route consistently, and watch for fever, which is the best indicator of many infections. Also assess pulse rate, blood pressure, and skin, along with mucous membranes, liver, spleen, and lymph nodes. Infection often increases pulse rate, but some infections decrease it. Assess blood pressure for hypotension in severe infections or when complications are possible. Record skin color, temperature, and turgor, and ask the patient about the presence of pruritus. Monitor for changes in any of these assessment parameters.

Chapter 2:
Bacterial
infections

1. b Meningococcal infections occur most commonly among children ages 6 months to 1 year. Sex of the child is not an issue; however, meningococcal infections are also prevalent among male military recruits (related to overcrowding). Although transmission is by carrier, the carrier population is not specific to school-age children or to those living in urban housing.

2. a Transmission of *N. meningitides* occurs through inhalation of an infected droplet from a carrier in up to 38% of the general population. Direct or indirect contact, enteric contamination of food, and vectors are not modes of transmission for these gram-negative bacteria.

3. b In suspected meningococcal infection, treatment includes aqueous penicillin G, ampicillin, or cephalosporins such as cefoxitin and moxalactam. Chloramphenicol is given I.V. if the patient is allergic to penicillins and related drugs. Minocycline is used for chemoprophylaxis of those in close contact with the patient and to temporarily eradicate the infection in carriers. To prevent the spread of meningococcal infections, respiratory isolation is imposed until the patient has received antibiotic therapy for 24 hours. Strict isolation is unnecessary. Delaying treatment until the infection is diagnosed places the patient at increased risk for complications.

4. c Unless treated promptly, fulminant meningococcemia is fatal in up to 20% of patients, causing respiratory or cardiac failure in 6 to 24 hours. Symptoms of all meningococcal infections result from tissue damage. A rare chronic form of meningococcemia is characterized by intermittent fever, joint pain, an enlarged spleen, and a maculopapular rash.

5. c Nontyphoidal salmonellosis generally follows ingestion of contaminated or inadequately processed foods, especially eggs, chicken, turkey, and duck. Proper cooking reduces the risk of contracting salmonellosis but doesn't eliminate it. Other means of contracting salmonellosis include contact with infected persons or animals (unlikely to affect a group of persons at the same time), and a contaminated water supply (likely to infect a larger population segment). Fecal-oral spread is more common among children under age 5.

6. d Salmonellosis is 20 times more common in patients with acquired immunodeficiency syndrome (AIDS) than among the general population. Specific features of salmonellosis in this population include an inability to identify the infection's source and a tendency for the infection to recur once antimicrobial therapy is discontinued. Enterocolitis and bacteremia are especially common (and more virulent) in AIDS patients and others at risk (infants, the elderly, and those weakened by other infections). Patients with chronic degenerative diseases are not at special risk for salmonellosis.

7. d When caring for a patient with salmonellosis, follow enteric precautions to prevent transmission of infection through direct and indirect contact with feces. Also use and teach patients proper hand-washing technique. Continue enteric precautions until three negative stool cultures are obtained—the first after 48 hours of antibiotic therapy, followed by two more at 24-hour intervals. Universal precautions are employed with *all* patients. Strict isolation prevents transmission of contagious or virulent organisms by air or contact. It requires a private room with a closed door; mask, gown, and gloves; special ventilation; and special procedures for handling contaminated products. Contact isolation prevents transmission of epidemiologically important infections that don't require strict isolation. Health care workers should wear masks, gowns, or gloves for direct or close contact, depending on the infection.

8. c Drainage in *Pseudomonas* infections has a distinct, sickly sweet odor and a greenish-blue pus that forms a crust on the infection site. None of the other color-odor combinations is specific to *Pseudomonas*.

9. a When assessing patients at high risk for septic shock, report any changes in mental status and urinary output promptly and respond with immediate volume expansion treatment. Sudden fever and chills may also appear in early septic shock, but urinary output changes are necessary to distinguish septic shock from other acute systemic infections. Tachycardia is also present in early septic shock. It is coupled with a full, bounding pulse rather than the weak, thready pulse that indicates hypovolemic shock. Hyperglycemia and thirst also appear in septic shock, but when they are coupled with hyperpnea, they are more likely to imply diabetic ketoacidosis.

10. b *Haemophilus influenzae* provokes a characteristic tissue response—acute suppurative inflammation, often with mucosal edema and a thick exudate. Lymph node tenderness and swelling and painful, suppurative buboes occur in bubonic plague. Pertussis causes a spasmodic, recurrent cough that ends with a loud, crowing inspiratory "whoop," giving the disease its common name, whooping cough. A thick, patchy, grayish-green membrane on mucous membranes of the pharynx, larynx, tonsils, and soft palate characterizes diphtheria.

Chapter 3: Viral infections

1. c Isolation of the influenza virus type from chicken embryos inoculated with nasal secretions from infected patients is essential at the first sign of an epidemic because early cases are often mistaken for other respiratory disorders. This is especially important because signs and symptoms are not pathognomonic. However, once an influenza epidemic is confirmed, observation of the clinical picture is sufficient for diagnosis. Serum antibody titers and nose and throat cultures help confirm the diagnosis in early cases. Uncomplicated cases exhibit decreased white blood cell (WBC) counts with an increase in lymphocytes, but this is not a specific diagnostic finding.

2. b A remarkable feature of the influenza virus is its capacity for antigenic variation. This is termed antigenic shift when a major change occurs that leads to pandemics. Antigenic drift is a minor change that occurs yearly or every few years. Type A and B viruses strike annually because of minor changes; new serotypes of type A cause epidemics every 3 years, whereas new serotypes of type B cause epidemics every 4 to 6 years. Type C is endemic and causes only sporadic cases.

3. b The incidence of influenza is highest in school-age children. However, its severity is greatest in the very young, the elderly, and those with chronic diseases.

4. a Fever that persists for longer than 3 to 5 days signals the onset of complications. Most symptoms subside within this time. However, cough and weakness may persist, with lack of energy and easy fatigability lasting for several weeks, especially in the elderly. Cervical adenopathy and croup may occur with influenza in children.

5. d Rodents are the reservoir for the hantavirus. The deer mouse is the primary reservoir, although it has also been found in piñon mice, brush mice, and western chipmunks. Known hantavirus infections that have been described in adults have been associated with activities that bring humans into contact with infected rodents. Such rodents manifest no apparent illness but shed the virus in feces, urine, and saliva. Transmission of hantavirus by mosquitoes, fleas, and other arthropods has not been reported. Dogs and cats are not natural carriers of this virus, and person-to-person transmission has not been associated with hantavirus infection.

6. a The most common findings on physical examination are an increased heart rate (generally equal to or greater than 120 beats/minute) and respiratory rate (generally 28 breaths/minute or more). Headache and myalgias are common, along with fever, cough, nausea, and vomiting. Patients typically progress to pulmonary edema associated with severe hypotension and cardiac arrest.

7. d Although only 65% of patients initially show chest X-ray abnormalities, 94% subsequently developed bilateral diffuse infiltrates (signs that are consistent with adult respiratory distress syndrome). Air in the pleural space, especially when accompanied by a mediastinal shift, confirms a pneumothorax. Patchy bilateral consolidation occurs with respiratory pneumonia. Upper lobe consolidation that causes bulging of fissures typically (but not always) occurs in *Klebsiella* pneumonia.

8. c The common cold, an acute, usually afebrile viral infection causing inflammation of the upper respiratory tract, accounts for more lost time from school and work than any other cause. Respiratory syncytial virus is the leading cause of lower respiratory tract infections in infants and young children. Adenoviruses cause acute, self-limiting febrile infections, with inflammation of the respiratory or ocular mucous membranes, or both. Influenza, an acute, highly contagious respiratory tract infection, occurs sporadically or in epidemics, with its highest incidence in school-age children.

9. d Varicella (chickenpox) calls for strict isolation until all vesicles and most of the scabs disappear (usually about 1 week after onset of the rash). Chickenpox is probably communicable from 1 day before lesions erupt to 6 days after vesicles form, although transmission is primarily by direct contact with respiratory secretions, and less often by contact with skin lesions. Children can return to school if just a few scabs remain because chickenpox is no longer contagious at this stage. The rash typically progresses from macules to papules to clear vesicles on an erythematous base. The vesicles become cloudy and break easily; then scabs form. New vesicles continue to develop for 3 to 4 days, so that the rash contains a combination of red papules, vesicles, and scabs in various stages.

10. d Indirect immunofluorescence, showing antibodies to Epstein-Barr virus and cellular antigens, is usually more definitive than heterophile antibodies (agglutinins for sheep red blood cells) in diagnosing infectious mononucleosis. WBC count and liver function changes support, but don't confirm, the diagnosis.

Chapter 4: Fungal infections

1. d The most common predisposing factor for candidiasis remains the use of broad-spectrum antibiotics. Other factors that can permit sudden proliferation of these fungi, which are part of the normal oral, GI, vaginal, and skin flora, include rising glucose levels from diabetes mellitus, lowered resistance from a disease such as cancer, immunosuppressive drug therapy or disease such as human immunodeficiency virus infection, radiation, aging, systemic introduction from I.V. or urinary catheters, drug abuse, total parenteral nutrition, and surgery.

2. b Systemic infections with candidiasis, though rare, are prevalent in hospitalized patients who are immunosuppressed or diabetic, and in drug abusers. Other hospitalized patients may also be at risk. Use of an I.V. or urinary catheter or other invasive device contaminated by the proliferating flora can also precipitate systemic infection. Age and antibiotic therapy do increase the risk, specifically for systemic candidiasis.

3. a Systemic infection produces high, spiking fever, chills, hypotension, prostration, myalgias, arthralgias, and rash. More specific symptoms depend on the infection site: If pulmonary, look for hemoptysis, cough, and fever; if renal, assess for fever, flank pain, dysuria, hematuria, pyuria, or cloudy urine; if the central nervous system is affected, check for headache, nuchal rigidity, seizures, and focal neurologic deficits; if the infection is endocardial, assess for systolic or diastolic murmurs, fever, chest pain, and embolic phenomena; and if the infection is ophthalmic, examine the patient for endophthalmitis, blurred vision, scotoma, and exudate.

4. d Treatment for systemic infections consists of I.V. amphotericin B or fluconazole. Clotrimazole, fluconazole, and miconazole are effective in treating superficial mucous membrane and vaginal *Candida* infections. Ketoconazole or fluconazole is the primary choice for chronic candidiasis of the mucous membranes.

5. c Allergic aspergillosis is an asthmatic reaction characterized by wheezing, dyspnea, cough with some sputum production, pleural pain, and fever. Aspergillosis endophthalmitis causes clouded vision, eye pain, and reddened conjunctivae. It eventually infects the anterior and posterior chambers, produces a purulent exudate, and leads to blindness. Aspergilloma may produce no symptoms, or mimic tuberculosis, causing a productive cough and purulent or blood-tinged sputum, dyspnea, empyema, and lung abscesses.

6. a *Aspergillus* is a fungus found worldwide, often in fermenting compost piles and damp hay. It's transmitted primarily through inhalation of fungal spores. In aspergillus endophthalmitis, spores invade a wound or other tissue injury. Ingestion and skin contamination are not modes of transmission. Culture of mouth scrapings or sputum may demonstrate the presence of *Aspergillus* even in healthy individuals, who may harbor this fungus without displaying overt signs of infection. Clinical infection occurs only when some factor or factors increase patient vulnerability to *Aspergillus*.

7. d Allergic aspergillosis requires desensitization and, possibly, steroid therapy. Treatment of aspergilloma involves local excision of the lesion and supportive therapy, such as chest physiotherapy and coughing, to improve pulmonary function. Disseminated aspergillosis and aspergillosis endophthalmitis require a 2- to 3-week course of I.V. amphotericin B (as well as prompt cessation of immunosuppressive therapy). Aspergillosis doesn't require isolation.

8. c Currently, patients with acquired immunodeficiency syndrome are the group most commonly infected with cryptococcosis, an asymptomatic pulmonary infection that disseminates to extrapulmonary sites. Other immunocompromised persons also at risk include those receiving immunosuppressants and those with Hodgkin's disease, sarcoidosis, leukemia, and lymphomas.

9. a Fatal disseminated histoplasmosis is most common in infants and elderly men. Other forms of histoplasmosis are more common in adult males, probably as the result of their occupational exposure to *Histoplasma capsulatum.* Adolescents and elderly females are not particularly at risk for histoplasmosis.

10. b Infuse I.V. amphotericin B slowly; too-rapid infusion may cause circulatory collapse. Despite slow infusion, you will need to monitor vital signs during infusion. The patient may develop a fever, which should subside within 1 to 2 hours. Watch for decreased urinary output and monitor laboratory studies for increased blood urea nitrogen and creatinine levels, and hypokalemia, which may indicate renal toxicity. Report any hearing loss, tinnitus, or dizziness immediately; these indicate ototoxicity. Relieve adverse effects with prescribed antiemetics and antipyretics.

Chapter 5:
Protozoal
infections

1. d *P. carinii* is part of the normal flora in most healthy persons, but becomes an aggressive pathogen in the immunocompromised patient. The organism exists as a saprophyte in the lungs of humans and various animals. However, the disease is not transmitted from person to person or from animals to humans. The primary transmission route seems to be air (although the organism resides in most people), not fomites adhering to articles.

2. a *Pneumocystis carinii* pneumonia (PCP) begins with increasing shortness of breath and a nonproductive cough. The patient may report anorexia, fatigue, and weight loss. Throughout the illness he may report a low-grade, intermittent fever. Although he may have hypoxemia and hypercapnea, he may fail to exhibit significant clinical symptoms. Cyanosis may appear with acute illness, depending on the hemoglobin level. Decreased breath sounds develop in patients with advanced pneumonia.

3. c Histologic studies confirm *P. carinii* infection. In many patients with HIV, initial examination of a first-morning sputum specimen may be sufficient. This is usually ineffective in HIV-negative patients. In all patients, fiber-optic bronchoscopy is most commonly used to confirm PCP. Transbronchial biopsy and open lung biopsy are less commonly used. A chest X-ray may show slowly progressing, fluffy infiltrates and occasional nodular lesions or a spontaneous pneumothorax. These findings must be differentiated from findings in other types of pneumonia or adult respiratory distress syndrome. A gallium scan may show increased uptake over the lungs even when the chest X-ray appears relatively normal.

4. a Leucovorin calcium (citrovorum factor or folinic acid), a reduced form of folic acid that is readily converted into other folic acids, may be used to reduce bone marrow suppression associated with co-trimoxazole therapy, and thus may be used prophylactically in patients with HIV infection. Folic acid (vitamin B_9), which is necessary for normal erythropoiesis and nucleoprotein synthesis, is used to treat megaloblastic anemia or macrocytic anemia secondary to folic acid deficiency. Cyanocobalamin (vitamin B_{12}), a coenzyme for various metabolic functions necessary for cell replication and hematopoiesis, is used to treat vitamin B_{12} deficiency caused by inadequate diet, subtotal gastrectomy, or other conditions or disorders. Pyridoxine hydrochloride (vitamin B_6), a coenzyme necessary for various metabolic functions and required for amino acid metabolism, is used to treat B_6 deficiency anemias and seizures. It is also used to prevent B_6 deficiency during isoniazid therapy.

5. d Trimetrexate glucuronate prevents reduction of folic acid to tetrahydrofolate by binding to dihydrofolate reductase. It has recently been approved as an alternative treatment for moderate to severe PCP. It may benefit patients who can't take co-trimoxazole due to adverse effects or poor response. Pentamidine isethionate is also used in PCP treatment. However, its I.V. form may cause toxic effects. The inhaled form, though well tolerated, may not effectively reach the lung apices. Vindesine sulfate arrests mitosis in metaphase, blocking cell division. It is used experimentally to treat acute lymphoblastic leukemia, breast cancer, malignant melanoma, lymphosarcoma, and non–small cell lung cancer.

6. c Because symptoms of malaria mimic other diseases, unequivocal diagnosis depends on laboratory identification of the parasites in red blood cells of peripheral blood smears. The Centers for Disease Control and Prevention can identify donors responsible for transfusion malaria through indirect fluorescent serum antibody tests. These tests are unreliable during the acute phase because antibodies can be undetectable for up to 2 weeks after onset. A history of travel to endemic areas, recent blood transfusion, or drug abuse in a person with high fever of unknown origin strongly suggests malaria and may prompt testing for parasite identification. Protein and leukocytes in urine sediment (not parasites) along with low hemoglobin and normal to decreased leukocyte counts support the diagnosis of malaria.

7. b Malaria is best treated with oral chloroquine in all but chloroquine-resistant *P. falciparum.* Chloroquine may be given I.M. if the patient is vomiting or comatose. Oral quinine is used to treat malaria due to *P. falciparum.* It is given for 10 days concurrently with pyrimethamine and a sulfonamide such as sulfadiazine. Primaquine phosphate is the only drug available in the United States that is effective against the hepatic stage of malaria. It is given daily for 2 weeks.

8. b *E. histolytica* is transmitted through ingesting feces-contaminated food or water. Airborne, contact, and vectorborne transmission are not implicated. Airborne transmission results from inhalation of contaminated aerosolized droplets. In contact transmission, the susceptible host comes into direct contact with the source or indirect contact with contaminated inanimate objects or fomites. Vectorborne transmission occurs when an intermediate carrier (vector), such as a flea or a mosquito, transfers an organism.

9. b Attachment of *G. lamblia* to the intestinal lumen causes superficial mucosal invasion and destruction, inflammation, and irritation. These changes affect food transit time through the small intestine and result in malabsorption, especially of fats and fat-soluble vitamins. Because the mucosal invasion is superficial, perforation and hemorrhage do not occur. Stools may contain mucus. Trophozoite attachment to the small bowel's epithelial surface also does not result in bowel obstruction.

10. d Treatment of toxoplasmosis is most effective during the acute stage and consists of sulfonamides and pyrimethamine. These are administered for about 4 weeks, sometimes with the addition of folinic acid to control pyrimethamine's adverse effects. A 10-day course of metronidazole is prescribed in giardiasis. Amebic dysentery may be treated with an amebicide, such as emetine hydrochloride in combination with tetracycline, which destroys intestinal bacteria on which the amoebae would feed. Iodoquinol is an effective amebicide for asymptomatic carriers of amebiasis.

Chapter 6: Helminthic infections

1. a Stage 1 invasion symptoms include all of the GI upsets Mr. Brown is experiencing. They occur 1 week after ingestion of uncooked or undercooked meat (such as pork) containing *T. spiralis* cysts. During this stage, the adult roundworm reproduces and releases larvae. During stage 2, dissemination, *T. spiralis* larvae penetrate the intestinal mucosa and begin to migrate to striated muscle, causing edema, muscle pain, and, occasionally, itching and burning skin, sweating, skin lesions, fever, and delirium. Stage 3—encystment—is marked by the invasion of muscle fibers by *T. spiralis* larvae, which then become encysted. Trichinosis has no stage 4.

2. c Gastric juices free the worm from the cyst capsule; it then reaches sexual maturity within a few days. Thorough cooking (internal temperature of 150° F [5.5° C] would kill the trichinae; lesser temperatures have no effect. Salivary juices and intestinal secretions don't dissolve the cyst.

3. c After the female roundworm burrows into the intestinal mucosa and reproduces, larvae are transmitted through the lymphatic system and bloodstream, becoming embedded as cysts in striated muscle in the diaphragm, chest, and extremities. Human-to-human transmission does not take place. Animals become infected by ingesting cysts (not larvae) in contaminated flesh. Invasion occurs via the GI tract; then larvae penetrate the mucosa to travel in body fluids.

4. b Thiabendazole effectively combats trichinae during the invasion (intestinal) stage. Severe infection may require the use of glucocorticoids to treat inflammation. Mebendazole is used to treat hookworm and roundworm infections because it blocks helminth nutrition. Piperazine is used as primary anti-*Ascaris* drug therapy, temporarily paralyzing the worms so that they can be expelled by peristalsis.

5. d Hookworm disease is transmitted to humans through direct skin penetration (usually in the foot) by hookworm larvae in soil contaminated with feces containing hookworm ova. Trichinosis and taeniasis (tapeworm disease) are transmitted to humans by ingestion of undercooked meats (or fish) containing encysted worms. Pinworms (enterobiasis) are transmitted directly (anus-hand-mouth) or indirectly from contact with contaminated bed linens and clothing.

6. b Hookworm larvae travel through the lymphatics to the pulmonary capillaries, where they penetrate alveoli and move up the bronchial tree to the trachea and epiglottis. They are swallowed and enter the GI tract. Trichinae travel through blood and lymphatic fluid from the intestinal mucosa to disseminate and encyst. Enterobiasis can be transmitted by direct hand contact, during which ova are transferred from the anus to the mouth. *Schistosoma* larvae penetrate skin or mucous membranes and travel to the hepatic portal circulation, where they mature. They then migrate to other parts of the body, laying eggs in blood vessels surrounding the large intestine or urinary bladder.

7. a Treatment for hookworm infection includes mebendazole or pyrantel and an iron-rich diet or iron supplements to prevent or correct anemia related to intestinal blood loss. Trichinosis may require fever-reducing measures. Ascariasis can result in intestinal obstruction, necessitating nasogastric suction. During treatment for pork tapeworm, laxatives and induced vomiting are contraindicated because of the danger of autoinfection.

8. b Tell the patient who will receive niclosamide therapy for taeniasis not to consume anything after midnight on the day treatment begins because the drug must be given on an empty stomach. Patients receiving sulfonamide drugs need to increase their oral fluid intake to help prevent crystal formation in the renal tubules. Patients being treated for schistosomiasis require reexamination in 3 to 6 months, with treatment resumed if living eggs are detected. Patients treated with thiabendazole for threadworm infection will need protein replacement, blood transfusions, and I.V. fluids.

9. c Before giving piperazine, obtain a history of seizure disorders. Piperazine may aggravate these disorders and is contraindicated in such a history. Piperazine is also contraindicated in patients with impaired renal or hepatic function. It should be used with caution in severely malnourished patients and those with anemia; the drug can cause hemolytic anemia. It should be stopped if significant GI reactions occur. It is not ototoxic, and does not adversely affect coagulation.

10. d Diagnosis of strongyloidiasis requires observation of *S. stercoralis* larvae in a fresh stool specimen because 2 hours after excretion, rhabdoid (rod-shaped) larvae look like hookworm larvae. Schistosomiasis is diagnosed by identifying ova in the urine or stool, with confirmation by mucosal lesion biopsy. Enterobiasis is diagnosed by identifying *Enterobus* ova recovered from the perianal area with a cellophane tape swab. Tapeworm disease is diagnosed by laboratory identification of ova or worm body segments in feces, and may require multiple specimens for confirmation.

Chapter 7: Miscellaneous infections

1. d Transmission of ornithosis to humans from infected birds occurs primarily through inhalation of dust containing *C. psittaci* from bird droppings. Less often, it may be transmitted through direct contact with infected secretions or body tissues. Person-to-person transmission is rare. The disease is mainly associated with occupational exposure to birds.

2. a Other signs and symptoms include abdominal distention and tenderness, nausea, vomiting, photophobia, decreased pulse rate, slightly increased respirations, secondary purulent rash, and a faint macular rash.

3. b Firm diagnosis of ornithosis requires recovery of *C. psittaci* from mice, eggs, or tissue culture inoculated with the patient's blood or sputum. Recovering the intracellular parasite from bird droppings, cultures, or cells is not definitive.

4. d Ornithosis calls for treatment with tetracycline. If the infection is severe, tetracycline may be administered I.V. until the fever subsides. Fever and other symptoms should begin to subside 48 to 72 hours after antibiotic treatment begins, but treatment must continue for 2 weeks after temperature returns to normal. If the patient can't tolerate tetracycline, penicillin G procaine or chloramphenicol may be substituted. Methicillin is not indicated for this disorder.

5. b Tampons are clearly implicated in toxic shock syndrome (TSS), although their exact role is unclear. This fits this patient's clinical picture, assuming that she is menstruating and uses tampon protection. If she is not menstruating, TSS may be linked to *S. aureus* infection associated with abscesses, osteomyelitis, and postsurgical infections, so these might become history concerns. Exposure via a personal contact or travel does not occur in TSS, and this patient's symptoms are not those of measles or German measles.

6. b TSS produces vaginal hyperemia and discharge, along with conjunctival hyperemia. Central nervous system effects include disorientation, without focal signs such as nuchal rigidity. Mild renal failure with elevated blood urea nitrogen and creatinine levels may occur, as well as oliguria related to hypovolemia. Anuria would not be expected.

7. c Within a few hours of TSS onset, a deep red rash develops— especially on the palms and soles—and later desquamates. Vesicular lesions on the labia or oropharynx occur in herpes simplex infection; vesicular lesions locally confined to one dermatome occur with herpes zoster. A macular rash starting on the face and then generalizing could be from rubella or rubeola, or from scarlet fever, exanthem subitum, or other similar infections.

8. c Treatment of TSS consists of I.V. antistaphylococcal antibiotics that are beta-lactamase-resistant, such as oxacillin or nafcillin. Ampicillin and amoxicillin are aminopenicillins. Adding sulbactam to ampicillin also inactivates bacterial beta-lactamase. Methicillin and dicloxacillin are penicillinase-resistant penicillins. Carbenicillin and mezlocillin are extended spectrum penicillins.

9. c Although uncommon, complications of Rocky Mountain spotted fever include disseminated intravascular coagulation, lobar pneumonia, pneumonitis, otitis media, parotitis, shock, and renal failure. A deer tick bite may cause Lyme disease. Rocky Mountain spotted fever is transmitted by the wood tick in the west and by the dog tick in the east. In addition, it can be acquired through inhalation or through contact of abraded skin with tick excreta or tissue juices. Generally, the shorter the incubation time, the more severe the infection. Rocky Mountain spotted fever is transmitted to a human by the prolonged bite (4 to 6 hours) of an adult tick.

10. a In Rocky Mountain spotted fever, treatment requires careful removal of the tick and administration of antibiotics, such as tetracycline or chloramphenicol, until 3 days after the fever subsides. Erythromycin is the drug of choice to treat Legionnaires' disease. Amantadine is an antiviral agent used to reduce the duration of influenza A infection. Amphotericin B is an antifungal agent used to treat such fungal infections as histoplasmosis.

Appendices and Index

Anti-Infective Drugs

For patients with infections, commonly prescribed drugs include antibacterial, antiviral, systemic antifungal, and antituberculin agents.

Antibacterial drugs

Aminoglycosides
Amikacin, gentamicin, kanamycin, neomycin, netilmicin, paromomycin, streptomycin, tobramycin

Indications
Severe gram-negative infections, such as septicemia, pneumonia, intra-abdominal infections, skin or bone infections, meningitis (requires intrathecal or intraventricular administration in addition to parenteral administration), and complicated urinary tract infections; used in combination with other antibiotics for infections caused by *Pseudomonas aeruginosa* and for endocarditis caused by enterococcus; may also be used as part of a multiple drug regimen for *Mycobacterium avium* complex infection in patients with AIDS.
• *Neomycin and kanamycin:* orally for hepatic encephalopathy and coma and for intestinal bacterial decontamination (preoperatively); topically for eye, ear, and skin infections (neomycin); kanamycin also used for peritoneal instillation during surgery and in other irrigation solutions
• *Paromomycin:* orally for intestinal amebiasis, hepatic coma, and parasitic infections
• *Streptomycin:* part of multidrug regimen for tuberculosis; also used for enterococcal endocarditis
• *Gentamicin and tobramycin:* administered as nebulizer therapy in respiratory tract infections (primarily associated with cystic fibrosis; efficacy has not been fully evaluated); also administered as impregnated beads imbedded into bone cement for gram-negative joint infections and orthopedic surgical procedures

Adverse reactions
• Blood: ***hemolytic anemia,*** leukopenia, ***thrombocytopenia*** (all rare)
• EENT: *ototoxicity* (vestibular and cochlear)
• GI: nausea, vomiting, diarrhea (uncommon)
• GU: ***nephrotoxicity*** (associated with serum trough levels above the normal therapeutic range; monitor serum drug levels and serum creatinine levels closely)
• Other: ***hypersensitivity,*** enhanced neuromuscular blockade

Carbapenems
Imipenem/cilastatin sodium

Indications
Serious infections caused by a wide range of susceptible gram-positive, gram-negative, and anaerobic bacteria; useful in mixed polymicrobial infections. Spectrum of activity includes *Pseudomonas aeruginosa.*

Adverse reactions
• Blood: eosinophilia, leukopenia, agranulocytosis, ***thrombocytopenia***
• CNS: *seizures* (with high doses or when dose has not been adjusted for renal dysfunction), dizziness, confusion, encephalopathy
• GI: nausea, vomiting, abdominal cramps, *pseudomembranous colitis*
• Other: ***hypersensitivity*** (rash, urticaria, pruritus, ***anaphylaxis***), superinfection, crossallergenicity between imipenem and penicillins

---

Common reactions are in *italics;* life-threatening reactions are in ***bold italics.***

Cephalosporins

- *First-generation cephalosporins:* cefadroxil, cefazolin, cephalexin, cephalothin, cephapirin, cephradine
- *Second-generation cephalosporins:* cefaclor, cefamandole, cefmetazole, cefonicid, ceforanide, cefotetan, cefoxitin, cefprozil, cefuroxime, loracarbef
- *Third-generation cephalosporins:* cefixime, cefoperazone, cefotaxime, cefpodoxime, ceftazidime, ceftizoxime, ceftriaxone

Indications

Infections of the skin, soft tissues, respiratory tract (bronchitis, pneumonia, otitis media, sinusitis), bones, joints, and urinary tract caused by a wide array of bacteria (susceptibilities depend on the generation of cephalosporin)

- *First-generation drugs:* most active against gram-positive bacteria; active against staphylococci, streptococci, *Escherichia coli, Klebsiella* species, and *Proteus mirabilis;* used prophylactically to reduce infections in patients undergoing surgical procedures (cardiac, orthopedic, gynecologic, GI); commonly used to treat skin or skin-structure infections
- *Second-generation drugs:* less activity than first-generation cephalosporins against gram-positive bacteria, but expanded activity to cover more gram-negative organisms, including some ampicillin-resistant strains of *Haemophilus influenzae* and *Moraxella (Branhamella) catarrhalis* that may cause upper respiratory tract infections such as bronchitis, sinusitis, and otitis media
- *Cefuroxime:* spectrum expanded to cover *Haemophilus influenzae*
- *Cefoxitin, cefotetan, cefmetazole:* spectrum expanded to include anaerobic organisms (such as *Bacteroides fragilis*); used for suspected intra-abdominal infections (peritonitis, abscess) and gynecologic infections
- *Third-generation drugs:* spectrum of activity expanded to cover more relatively resistant gram-negative bacteria, such as *Serratia, Citrobacter, Enterobacter,* and others that are associated with nosocomial infections but varies with each third-generation cephalosporin; possess the least activity of the three generations against gram-positive bacteria; penetration into cerebrospinal fluid allows use in meningitis; also used for cervical and urethral gonorrhea caused by *Neisseria gonorrhoeae* and for serious Lyme disease
- *Ceftazidime:* serious infections caused by *Pseudomonas aeruginosa* (often in combination with aminoglycosides)

Adverse reactions

- Blood: eosinophilia, reversible neutropenia or leukopenia, **hemolytic anemia, thrombocytopenia**
- CNS: *seizures* (at high doses)
- GI: *nausea, vomiting, diarrhea,* dyspepsia, cholestasis (ceftriaxone), **pseudomembranous colitis** (toxicogenic *Clostridium difficile* diarrhea)
- GU: **nephrotoxicity** (rare), transient elevated blood urea nitrogen
- Hepatic: elevated liver function test results
- Local: *phlebitis at I.V. site, pain at I.M. site*
- Other: **hypersensitivity** (rash, urticaria, **Stevens-Johnson syndrome, anaphylaxis**), bacterial and fungal superinfection, disulfuram-type reactions (only with cefamandole, cefoperazone, cefotetan, and cefmetazole)

Fluoroquinolones

Ciprofloxacin, enoxacin, lomefloxacin, norfloxacin, ofloxacin

Indications

Infections of the respiratory tract (excluding *Streptococcus pneumoniae* pneumonia), skin, soft tissue, bones, or joints; urinary tract infections (including prostatitis); sexually transmitted disease (gonococcal and nongonococcal urethritis or cervicitis); and infectious diarrhea; has an extended spectrum of activity against gram-positive and gram-negative bacteria compared with other oral antibiotics; because of broad spectrum of activity, may be an appropriate choice for early conversion from I.V. to oral anti-infective therapy

Adverse reactions

- CNS: dizziness, headache, *seizures*

Common reactions are in *italics;* life-threatening reactions are in **bold italics.**

• GI: *nausea, vomiting, diarrhea, abdominal pain*
• Skin: rash, urticaria, pruritus, photosensitivity, *anaphylaxis*

Macrolides
Azithromycin, clarithromycin, erythromycin, troleandomycin

Indications
Respiratory, genital, GI tract, and skin or soft-tissue infections caused by susceptible gram-positive (*Streptococcus, Staphylococcus*) and "atypical" organisms (*Chlamydia, Mycoplasma, Legionella*). Azithromycin and clarithromycin extend coverage to *Haemophilus influenzae* and *Moraxella (Branhamella) catarrhalis.* Useful in community-acquired pneumonia. Also used in Lyme disease, pelvic inflammatory disease, primary syphilis (if the patient is allergic to penicillin), and as an alternative to tetracycline in nongonococcal urethritis or cervicitis.

Adverse reactions
• GI: *nausea,* vomiting, *diarrhea,* abdominal pain (especially with erythromycin)
• Hepatic: hepatic dysfunction, cholestatic hepatitis (erythromycin estolate)
• Local: *phlebitis or pain at I.V. site* (only erythromycin is administered parenterally)
• Other: fever, superinfection, *hypersensitivity* (urticaria, skin eruptions, rash, *anaphylaxis*), ototoxicity (with high I.V. doses and renal or hepatic dysfunction)

Monobactams
Aztreonam

Indications
Serious infections caused by gram-negative bacteria, including susceptible strains of *Pseudomonas aeruginosa.* Aztreonam has a narrow spectrum of activity against aerobic gram-negative bacteria, similar to that of the aminoglycosides.

Adverse reactions
• Blood: pancytopenia, anemia, neutropenia, *thrombocytopenia*

• CNS: *seizures* (rare)
• GI: nausea, vomiting, abdominal cramps, diarrhea, *pseudomembranous colitis*
• Local: phlebitis at I.V. site, *pain at I.M. site*
• Other: *hypersensitivity* (rash, urticaria, pruritus, *anaphylaxis*)

Penicillins
Natural penicillins, aminopenicillins, extended-spectrum penicillins, penicillinase-resistant penicillins

Natural penicillins
Penicillin G benzathine, penicillin G potassium, penicillin G procaine, penicillin G sodium, penicillin V potassium

Indications
Infections caused by susceptible strains of gram-positive bacteria, such as *Streptococcus pneumoniae;* groups A, B, C, D (nonenterococcal), and G streptococci; and *Streptococcus viridans;* infections caused by *Bacillus anthracis, Corynebacterium diphtheriae, Listeria monocytogenes,* and anaerobic mouth flora, such as *Peptostreptococcus* and *Fusobacterium*

Adverse reactions
(for all penicillins)
• Blood: **hemolytic anemia,** neutropenia, leukopenia, **thrombocytopenia,** increased bleeding time (extended-spectrum penicillins)
• CNS: agitation, confusion, myoclonus, *seizures* (with high doses or when dose has not been adjusted for renal impairment)
• GI: *nausea, vomiting, epigastric distress, diarrhea* (most common with ampicillin and amoxicillin or clavulanic acid), *pseudomembranous colitis*
• GU: interstitial nephritis
• Hepatic: elevated liver function test results
• Metabolic: hyperkalemia (penicillin G potassium), hypokalemia and hypernatremia (extended-spectrum penicillins and penicillin G sodium)
• Local: *phlebitis at I.V. site, pain at I.M. site*
• Other: *hypersensitivity* (rash, urticaria, fever, severe dermatitis, laryngospasm, angioneurotic edema, *anaphylaxis*)

Common reactions are in *italics;* life-threatening reactions are in ***bold italics.***

Aminopenicillins
Amoxicillin, ampicillin, bacampicillin

Indications
Infections of the respiratory tract (pharyngitis, sinusitis, bronchitis, pneumonia), urinary tract, skin, soft tissue, bones, or joints; gonococcal infections (most *Neisseria gonorrhoeae* strains are resistant); endocarditis; *Listeria* infections; otitis media; Lyme disease; septicemia; and meningitis caused by susceptible organisms. Less activity against gram-positive organisms compared with natural penicillins; however, the antibacterial spectrum is broadened to include *Escherichia coli, Haemophilus influenzae* (many strains are resistant), *Proteus mirabilis, Salmonella,* and *Shigella.*

Extended-spectrum penicillins
Azlocillin, carbenicillin, carbenicillin indanyl sodium, mezlocillin, piperacillin, ticarcillin; products available in combination with a beta-lactamase inhibitor include ampicillin/sulbactam, piperacillin/tazobactam, and ticarcillin/clavulanate potassium

Indications
Hospital-acquired pneumonia, septicemia, abdominal infections, fever with neutropenia, and urinary tract or gynecologic infections caused by a broad range of gram-positive, gram-negative, and anaerobic organisms; antibacterial spectrum broadened to include relatively resistant gram-negative and a few anaerobic organisms; however, provide less activity against gram-positive organisms than natural penicillins
• *Carbenicillin indanyl sodium:* urinary tract infections only; does not achieve adequate serum levels to be used for systemic infections (available as tablet only)

Penicillinase-resistant penicillins
Cloxacillin, dicloxacillin, methicillin, nafcillin, oxacillin

Indications
Systemic infections caused by penicillinase-producing staphylococci

Sulfonamides
Single agents: sulfacetamide, sulfacytine, sulfadiazine, sulfamethizole, sulfamethoxazole, sulfapyridine, sulfasalazine, sulfisoxazole
Combination products: co-trimoxazole (sulfamethoxazole-trimethoprim), erythromycin-sulfisoxazole

Indications
• *Single agents:* urinary tract infections, otitis media, nocardiosis, toxoplasmosis (with pyrimethamine), chancroid, and topically for skin and soft-tissue infections
• *Combination products:* otitis media due to gram-positive bacteria, *Haemophilus influenzae,* or *Moraxella (Branhamella) catarrhalis.* Co-trimoxazole is effective against a broad spectrum of bacteria and is useful in urinary tract infections, bronchitis, traveler's diarrhea, and *Pneumocystis carinii* pneumonia in patients with AIDS.

Adverse reactions
• Blood: **agranulocytosis, aplastic anemia, hemolytic anemia,** megaloblastic anemia, neutropenia, leukopenia, ***thrombocytopenia***
• CNS: headache, dizziness, insomnia
• GI: *anorexia, nausea, vomiting, abdominal pain, diarrhea,* **pseudomembranous colitis** (rare)
• GU: crystalluria (can lead to renal damage, hematuria)
• Other: tinnitus, ***hypersensitivity*** (rash, pruritus, skin eruptions, ***erythema multiforme [Stevens-Johnson syndrome],*** *fever,* serum sickness, ***anaphylaxis***)

Tetracyclines
Demeclocycline, doxycycline, minocycline, oxytetracycline, tetracycline

Indications
Lyme disease (tetracycline only), endemic typhus, chancroid, and infections caused by *Chlamydia* (nongonococcal urethritis or cervicitis, atypical pneumonia), *Mycoplasma* (atypical pneumonia), *Rickettsia* (Rocky Mountain spotted fever), and other uncom-

Common reactions are in *italics;* life-threatening reactions are in **bold italics.**

mon organisms; used in acute exacerbations of chronic bronchitis and systemic treatment of acne; effective against a relatively broad spectrum of gram-positive and gram-negative activity, although resistance can occur
• *Demeclocycline:* hyponatremia due to syndrome of inappropriate antidiuretic hormone
• *Minocycline:* asymptomatic carriers of *Neisseria meningitidis* when rifampin is contraindicated

Adverse reactions
• Blood: neutropenia, **thrombocytopenia, hemolytic anemia** (all rare)
• CNS: light-headedness, vertigo, pseudotumor cerebri (rare in infants)
• GI: anorexia, *nausea, vomiting, diarrhea,* **pancreatitis,** esophagitis, enterocolitis
• GU: blood urea nitrogen increase
• Hepatic: elevated liver function test results, **hepatotoxicity** (rare)
• Local: phlebitis at I.V. site, *pain at I.M. site*
• Skin: *photosensitivity, rash, urticaria*
• Other: dysphasia, glossitis, **hypersensitivity,** tooth discoloration

Miscellaneous antibacterial drugs

Chloramphenicol

Indications
Serious infections caused by susceptible bacteria resistant to other agents or when other agents are contraindicated (for example, penicillin or cephalosporin allergy); drug of choice for typhoid fever *(Salmonella typhosa).* Excellent CNS penetration allows use in meningitis; anaerobic activity allows use in brain abscess. Can be used in rickettsial infections (Rocky Mountain spotted fever)

Adverse reactions
• Blood: *aplastic anemia* (irreversible and not dose-related), hypoplastic anemia, **granulocytopenia,** thrombocytopenia (dose-related, reversible)
• CNS: headache, mild depression, confusion, delirium, peripheral neuropathy, optic neuritis (with prolonged therapy)

• CV: **gray syndrome in neonates** (abdominal distention, gray cyanosis, vasomotor collapse, respiratory distress, death due to accumulation of chloramphenicol)
• GI: nausea, vomiting, stomatitis, diarrhea, enterocolitis
• Other: jaundice, **hypersensitivity** (fever, rash, angioedema, **anaphylaxis**)

Clindamycin, lincomycin

Indications
Infections due to gram-positive (*Staphylococcus, Streptococcus*) or anaerobic (*Bacteroides fragilis*) organisms; particularly effective in infections caused by a mixture of these organisms, such as respiratory tract infections (aspiration pneumonia, empyema, lung abscess), intra-abdominal infections, skin and soft-tissue infections (diabetes-related foot ulcer), and pelvic inflammatory infections; lincomycin generally less active than clindamycin

Adverse reactions
• Blood: *leukopenia, neutropenia,* eosinophilia, **thrombocytopenia**
• CV: **hypotension, syncope, cardiac arrest after rapid I.V. administration** (all with lincomycin)
• GI: *nausea,* vomiting, abdominal pain, *diarrhea,* **pseudomembranous colitis** (due to *Clostridium difficile*), esophagitis, metallic taste
• Local: phlebitis at I.V. site, *pain and sterile abscess at I.M. site*
• Other: **hypersensitivity** (maculopapular rash, urticaria, **erythema multiforme,** generalized morbilliform rash, **anaphylaxis**)

Metronidazole

Indications
Anaerobic bacteria and many protozoa; indicated for serious infections such as intra-abdominal infections (peritonitis, abscess), gynecologic infections (trichomoniasis and *Gardnerella),* bone and joint infections, lower respiratory tract infections, CNS infections,

Common reactions are in *italics;* life-threatening reactions are in **bold italics.**

and septicemia; administered orally for pseudomembranous colitis associated with *Clostridium difficile*

Adverse reactions
• Blood: transient leukopenia, neutropenia
• CNS: *vertigo, headache, ataxia, incoordination, depression, restlessness, insomnia, sensory neuropathy, neuromyopathy, **seizures***
• GI: *nausea, vomiting, anorexia,* abdominal cramping, epigastric distress, metallic taste
• GU: darkened urine, polyuria, dysuria, incontinence
• Local: *thrombophlebitis after I.V. infusion*
• Other: hypersensitivity (urticaria, rash, pruritus), mutagenic and carcinogenic in mice (effects on humans not fully known)

Vancomycin

Indications
Gram-positive infections when bacteria are not susceptible to penicillins or when patient is allergic to penicillin; effective against *Streptococcus, Staphylococcus,* and *Corynebacterium;* major uses: resistant staphylococcal infections, enterococcal endocarditis, and orally to treat pseudomembranous colitis caused by *Clostridium difficile*

Adverse reactions
• Blood: neutropenia, ***thrombocytopenia***
• GU: ***nephrotoxicity***
• Local: pain or thrombophlebitis at I.V. site
• Skin: "red-neck" syndrome with rapid I.V. infusion (hypotension associated with a maculopapular rash on face, neck, trunk, and extremities)
• Other: *chills, fever,* **anaphylaxis,** superinfection, tinnitus, ototoxicity

Antiviral drugs

Acyclovir

Indications
• Parenterally for initial and recurrent mucosal or cutaneous herpes simplex virus types I and II in immunocompromised pa-

tients, severe first episodes of genital herpes infection, encephalitis caused by herpes simplex in patients over age 6 months, and varicella-zoster (chicken pox) infections in immunocompromised adults and children
• Orally for initial and recurrent genital herpes in selected patients and for acute treatment of herpes zoster (shingles) and varicella-zoster infections in patients under age 2
• Topically for mucocutaneous herpes simplex infections

Adverse reactions
• CNS: *headache; encephalopathic changes,* including lethargy, obtundation, tremor, confusion, hallucinations, agitation, ***seizures, coma*** (with I.V. dosage)
• CV: hypotension
• GI: *nausea, vomiting,* diarrhea
• GU: *increased blood urea nitrogen or serum creatinine levels,* renal dysfunction (especially with rapid I.V. infusion)
• Local: *inflammation, phlebitis, and irritation at injection site*
• Skin: rash, urticaria

Amantadine, rimantidine

Indications
Prophylaxis and symptomatic treatment of influenza A viral infections (not effective against influenza B infections); must be administered within 48 hours of onset of symptoms

Adverse reactions
• CNS: *irritability, insomnia,* anxiety, impaired concentration (all less common with rimantadine)
• CV: orthostatic hypotension, peripheral edema, ***congestive heart failure***
• GI: anorexia, nausea
• Skin: *livedo reticularis* (with prolonged use)

Didanosine

Indications
HIV infections when patient is unresponsive to or cannot tolerate zidovudine

Common reactions are in *italics;* life-threatening reactions are in **bold italics.**

Adverse reactions
- CNS: *headache, peripheral neuropathy,* asthenia, insomnia, CNS depression, seizures
- GI: *diarrhea, nausea, vomiting, abdominal pain,* constipation, stomatitis, taste loss or change, ***pancreatitis*** (can be severe)
- Hepatic: ***hepatotoxicity***
- Skin: rash, pruritus, alopecia
- Other: myalgia, arthritis, pain, cough, infection

Foscarnet

Indications
Cytomegalovirus retinitis in patients with AIDS

Adverse reactions
- Blood: anemia, ***bone marrow suppression*** (rare)
- CNS: *headache, fatigue, rigors, dizziness, hypoesthesia, paresthesia,* ***coma,*** visual field deficits, extrapyramidal reactions, ***cerebral edema***
- EENT: visual abnormalities
- GI: anorexia, *nausea, vomiting, diarrhea, abdominal pain,* **pancreatitis**
- GU: ***nephrotoxicity*** (in 30% of patients), ***acute renal failure***
- Respiratory: *cough, dyspnea,* ***bronchospasm***
- Skin: *rash, sweating*
- Other: fever, mineral and electrolyte disturbances (calcium, magnesium, potassium, phosphorus)

Ganciclovir

Indications
Cytomegalovirus (CMV) retinitis in immunocompromised patients; other CMV infections (pneumonia, GI infection) in immunosuppressed patients; prevention of CMV infection in transplant patients

Adverse reactions
- Blood: ***granulocytopenia, thrombocytopenia,*** anemia
- CNS: ataxia, dizziness, headache, confusion, seizures
- CV: arrhythmias, hypotension, hypertension
- GI: nausea, vomiting, diarrhea
- Hepatic: elevated liver function test results
- Local: erythema, pain, and phlebitis at injection site

Ribavirin

Indications
Severe lower respiratory tract infection due to respiratory syncytial virus in infants and children

Adverse reactions
- Blood: anemia, reticulocytosis
- CV: hypotension, ***cardiac arrest***
- EENT: conjunctivitis, eyelid rash or erythema
- Respiratory: worsening respiratory status
- Other: rash

Vidarabine

Indications
Herpes simplex encephalitis, neonatal herpes simplex infections, and herpes zoster in immunocompromised patients

Adverse reactions
- Blood: anemia, neutropenia, ***thrombocytopenia***
- CNS: tremor, dizziness, hallucinations, confusion, ataxia
- GI: anorexia, nausea, vomiting, diarrhea
- Skin: rash, pruritus

Zalcitabine

Indications
Advanced HIV infection; drug given with zidovudine

Common reactions are in *italics;* life-threatening reactions are in ***bold italics.***

Adverse reactions

- Blood: **bone marrow depression, granulocytopenia, thrombocytopenia**
- CNS: *peripheral neuropathy,* headache, fatigue
- GI: stomatitis, nausea, dysphagia, diarrhea
- Hepatic: elevated liver function test results
- Skin: rash, pruritus
- Other: myalgia, arthralgia, night sweats, fever, *pancreatitis*

Zidovudine

Indications
Orally for patients with symptomatic or asymptomatic HIV infections who have had two consecutive CD4+ T-cell counts of 500/mm³ or less

Adverse reactions
- Blood: **severe bone marrow depression, granulocytopenia, thrombocytopenia, thrombocytosis,** anemia
- CNS: *headache, malaise,* fatigue, confusion, insomnia, seizures
- GI: *nausea,* abdominal pain, diarrhea, vomiting
- Hepatic: elevated liver function test results
- Skin: *rash*
- Other: myalgia, fever, necrotizing myopathy

Systemic antifungal drugs

Amphotericin B

Indications
CNS (may require intrathecal injection in addition to I.V. administration), pulmonary, hepatic, renal, and other systemic fungal infections; blastomycosis, histoplasmosis, cryptococcosis, candidiasis, sporotrichosis, aspergillosis, phycomycosis (mucormycosis), and coccidioidomycosis

Adverse reactions
- Blood: anemia (normochromic, normocytic)
- CNS: headache, peripheral neuropathy
- CV: hypotension, arrhythmias, asystole

- GI: *anorexia, weight loss, nausea,* vomiting, abdominal pain
- GU: **nephrotoxicity** (in 80% of patients)
- Local: *thrombophlebitis, pain at injection site*
- Metabolic: hypokalemia, hypomagnesemia
- Other: *fever, chills,* myalgia, arthralgia
(*Note:* Risk of fever, chills, nausea, vomiting, and myalgia may be minimized by pretreating patient with antihistamines, antiemetics, and antipyretics.)

Fluconazole, itraconazole, ketoconazole

Indications
- *Fluconazole:* oropharyngeal, esophageal, and systemic candidiasis; cryptococcal meningitis (including prophylaxis in AIDS patients)
- *Itraconazole:* orally for systemic blastomycosis and histoplasmosis (includes HIV-positive patients)
- *Ketoconazole:* some systemic fungal infections, recalcitrant cutaneous dermatophyte infections, oral and esophageal candidiasis

Adverse reactions
- CNS: headache
- GI: nausea, vomiting, diarrhea
- Hepatic: **hepatotoxicity** (rarely, fatal), elevated liver enzyme levels (both with ketoconazole)
- Skin: rash, **Stevens-Johnson syndrome** (with fluconazole; rare)

Flucytosine

Indications
Serious infections caused by *Candida, Cryptococcus* (including meningitis); usually administered with amphotericin B for systemic fungal infections because of rapid development of resistance when flucytosine is used alone; can be used as monotherapy for fungal urinary tract infections

---

Common reactions are in *italics;* life-threatening reactions are in **bold italics.**

Adverse reactions
- Blood: anemia, ***bone marrow suppression, aplastic anemia,*** pancytopenia, ***thrombocytopenia***
- CNS: dizziness, drowsiness, confusion, headache, vertigo
- GI: *nausea, vomiting, diarrhea*
- Metabolic: elevated blood urea nitrogen, serum creatinine, and serum alkaline phosphatase levels
- Skin: rash, pruritus

Griseofulvin

Indications
Tinea infections of skin, nails, and hair that do not respond to topical agents. Because griseofulvin is not effective against other fungal infections, the organism should be identified as a dermatophyte before therapy is initiated.

Adverse reactions
- CNS: headache (early in treatment), transient decrease in hearing, fatigue (with large doses), mental confusion, psychoses, dizziness, insomnia, paresthesia (hands, feet)
- GI: nausea, vomiting, excessive thirst, diarrhea
- Skin: rash, urticaria, photosensitivity
- Other: estrogen-like effects in children, thrush

Miconazole

Indications
Systemic fungal infections (coccidioidomycosis, candidiasis, cryptococcosis, and paracoccidioidomycosis); topically for vaginal and other cutaneous fungal infections

Adverse reactions
- CNS: dizziness, drowsiness
- CV: tachycardia, arrhythmias
- GI: *nausea, vomiting,* diarrhea
- Local: *phlebitis at injection site*
- Skin: *pruritic rash*
- Other: fever, chills

Nystatin

Indications
Oral, GI, and vaginal (topical) infections (such as thrush) caused by *Candida albicans* and other candidal organisms

Adverse reactions
- GI: transient nausea, vomiting, diarrhea (usually with large oral doses)
- Skin: contact dermatitis (topical)

Antituberculins

Capreomycin

Indications
Tuberculosis (usually as part of a multidrug regimen)

Adverse reactions
- Blood: eosinophilia, leukocytosis, leukopenia
- CNS: headache, ***neuromuscular blockade***
- GU: ***nephrotoxicity***
- Other: *ototoxicity* (cranial nerve VIII)

Cycloserine

Indications
Tuberculosis (usually as part of a multidrug regimen)

Adverse reactions
- CNS: drowsiness, headache, vertigo, confusion, psychoses, ***seizures,*** *nervousness, hallucinations, depression*
- Other: rash

Ethambutol

Indications
Tuberculosis (usually as part of a multidrug regimen)

Common reactions are in *italics;* life-threatening reactions are in ***bold italics.***

Adverse reactions
- CNS: headache, dizziness, mental confusion
- EENT: optic neuritis
- GI: anorexia, nausea, vomiting
- Metabolic: elevated uric acid levels, precipitation of gout
- Other: *anaphylaxis,* fever, malaise

Ethionamide

Indications
Tuberculosis (usually as part of a multidrug regimen)

Adverse reactions
- CNS: depression, asthenia, *peripheral neuritis*
- GI: *anorexia, epigastric distress,* nausea, vomiting
- Hepatic: elevated liver function test results, hepatitis
- Skin: rash, *exfoliative dermatitis*

Isoniazid

Indications
Tuberculosis (usually as part of a multidrug regimen); may be used alone for prophylaxis (6 months to a year) in patients with a significant reaction to the Mantoux test

Adverse reactions
- Blood: *agranulocytosis, hemolytic anemia, aplastic anemia, thrombocytopenia,* leukopenia, neutropenia, eosinophilia
- CNS: *peripheral neuropathy* (preventable by using pyridoxine during isoniazid therapy)
- GI: nausea, vomiting, epigastric distress
- Hepatic: *hepatitis* (may be severe or fatal; highest incidence in individuals over age 35)
- Other: *hypersensitivity* (fever, skin eruptions)

Pyrazinamide

Indications
Tuberculosis (usually as part of a multidrug regimen)

Adverse reactions
- GI: anorexia, nausea, vomiting, diarrhea
- Hepatic: *hepatotoxicity*
- Metabolic: *hyperuricemia;* occasionally, precipitation of gout
- Other: fever, myalgia, arthralgia

Rifampin

Indications
Tuberculosis (usually as part of a multidrug regimen); also used to treat staphylococcal infections in combination with other antibiotics, for prophylaxis in persons exposed to *Haemophilus influenzae* type B infections, and to eradicate *Neisseria meningitidis* from the nasopharynx of asymptomatic carriers

Adverse reactions
- Blood: eosinophilia, transient leukopenia, *thrombocytopenia, hemolytic anemia*
- CNS: headache, fatigue, *drowsiness,* ataxia, dizziness
- GI: anorexia, nausea, vomiting, abdominal pain, diarrhea
- Hepatic: *hepatotoxicity,* transient elevations in liver function test results
- Skin: rash, urticaria
- Other: flulike syndrome, discoloration of body fluids (red-orange tears, feces, urine, sputum, sweat)

Drugs for AIDS infections

Atovaquone

Indications
Mild to moderate *Pneumocystis carinii* pneumonia in patients who can't tolerate co-trimoxazole

Adverse reactions
- CNS: *headache, insomnia,* asthenia, dizziness
- GI: *nausea, vomiting, diarrhea,* constipation
- Skin: *rash,* pruritus
- Other: *fever,* thrush

Common reactions are in *italics;* life-threatening reactions are in *__bold italics.__*

Co-trimoxazole

Indications
Treatment or prophylaxis of *P. carinii* pneumonia

Adverse reactions
- Blood: *agranulocytosis, hemolytic anemia,* megaloblastic anemia, neutropenia, leukopenia, *thrombocytopenia*
- CNS: headache, dizziness, tinnitus, insomnia
- GI: *nausea, vomiting, diarrhea,* abdominal pain, pseudomembranous colitis (rare)
- GU: *toxic nephrosis with oliguria and anuria,* crystalluria, hematuria, increased serum creatinine levels
- Skin: rash, pruritus, *skin eruptions,* **erythema multiforme (Stevens-Johnson syndrome), epidermal necrolysis, exfoliative dermatitis,** photosensitivity
- Other: *hypersensitivity* (fever, serum sickness, **anaphylaxis**)

Dapsone

Indications
Treatment or prophylaxis of *P. carinii* pneumonia; used in combination with trimethoprim for treatment; for prophylaxis, may be used as monotherapy or in combination with trimethoprim or pyrimethamine

Adverse reactions
- Blood: *aplastic anemia, agranulocytosis, hemolytic anemia* (especially in patients with glucose-6-phosphate dehydrogenase deficiency), methemoglobinemia, cyanosis
- CNS: insomnia, psychosis, headache, dizziness, severe malaise, paresthesia
- EENT: tinnitus, allergic rhinitis
- GI: anorexia, nausea, vomiting
- Hepatic: hepatitis, cholestatic jaundice
- Skin: rash

Pentamidine

Indications
Treatment or prophylaxis of *P. carinii* pneumonia

Adverse reactions
- Blood: *leukopenia, thrombocytopenia,* anemia
- CV: *hypotension,* orthostatic hypotension, tachycardia, arrhythmias
- Endocrine: *hypoglycemia,* hyperglycemia, hypocalcemia, *pancreatitis*
- GI: nausea, anorexia, metallic taste
- GU: *elevated serum creatinine levels,* renal failure, *nephrotoxicity* (in 25% of patients)
- Skin: rash, facial flushing, pruritus

Primaquine

Indications
Treatment or prophylaxis of *P. carinii* pneumonia in combination with clindamycin

Adverse reactions
- Blood: *hemolytic anemia* (in glucose-6-phosphate dehydrogenase deficiency), leukopenia, leukocytosis, mild anemia, *agranulocytosis* (rare), methemoglobinemia
- GI: nausea, vomiting, diarrhea, abdominal cramps
- Skin: urticaria
- Other: headache, disturbances of visual accommodation

Pyrimethamine

Indications
Toxoplasmosis in combination with sulfadiazine or clindamycin; prophylaxis of *P. carinii* pneumonia in combination with dapsone (second-line choice)

Adverse reactions
- Blood: *agranulocytosis, aplastic anemia,* megaloblastic anemia, *bone marrow suppression,* leukopenia, *thrombocytopenia,*

Common reactions are in *italics;* life-threatening reactions are in ***bold italics.***

pancytopenia, depletion of folic acid stores
• CNS: stimulation and *seizures* (acute toxicity)
• GI: anorexia, vomiting, diarrhea, atrophic glossitis
• Skin: rash, *erythema multiforme, toxic epidermal necrolysis*

Rifabutin

Indications
Prevention of disseminated *Mycobacterium avium* complex in patients with advanced HIV infection (CD4 + T-cell count less than 100/mm^3)

Adverse reactions
• Blood: neutropenia, leukopenia, *thrombocytopenia,* eosinophilia
• GI: dyspepsia, eructation, flatulence, nausea, vomiting, abdominal pain
• GU: *discolored urine*
• Skin: rash
• Other: uveitis, fever, myalgia, myositis, taste distortion

Sulfadiazine

Indications
Adjunctive treatment of toxoplasmosis

Adverse reactions
• Blood: *agranulocytosis, aplastic anemia,* megaloblastic anemia, *thrombocytopenia,* leukopenia, *hemolytic anemia*
• CNS: headache, mental depression, seizures, hallucinations
• GI: nausea, vomiting, diarrhea, abdominal pain, anorexia, stomatitis
• GU: *toxic nephrosis* with oliguria and anuria, crystalluria, hematuria
• Skin: urticaria, pruritus, photosensitivity, *erythema multiforme, skin eruptions, epidermal necrolysis, exfoliative dermatitis*
• Other: jaundice, *hypersensitivity (serum sickness, fever, anaphylaxis)*

Trimetrexate

Indications
Moderate to severe cases of *P. carinii* pneumonia in patients intolerant of or refractory to co-trimoxazole therapy. (*Note:* Leucovorin must be used daily throughout trimetrexate therapy and for 72 hours after discontinuation of this drug.)

Adverse reactions
• Blood: neutropenia, *thrombocytopenia*
• Skin: rash
• Other: *hepatotoxicity,* peripheral neuropathy

ICD-9-CM Classification of Infectious Disorders

The *International Classification of Diseases, 9th revision, Clinical Modification (ICD-9-CM)*, standardizes the classification of communicable or transmissible diseases and diseases of unknown but possibly infectious origin. Categories for *late effects* of infectious and parasitic diseases are grouped from **137** to **139**. *Acute respiratory infections* are categorized from **460** to **466**, and certain *localized infections* and *influenza* are categorized in the **487.0** to **487.8** series.

Diseases related to a *carrier or a suspected carrier of infectious organisms* are categorized from **V02.0** to **V02.9**.

Diseases coded **001** through **139** are organized as follows:
• **001** to **009**: Intestinal infectious diseases— excluding helminthiases (**120** to **129**)
• **010** to **018**: Tuberculosis
• **020** to **027**: Zoonotic bacterial diseases
• **030** to **041**: Other bacterial diseases
• **042** to **044**: Human immunodeficiency virus (HIV) infection
• **045** to **049**: Poliomyelitis and other nonarthropod-borne viral diseases of the central nervous system (CNS)
• **050** to **057**: Viral diseases accompanied by exanthem
• **060** to **066**: Arthropod-borne viral diseases
• **070** to **079**: Other diseases due to viruses and chlamydiae
• **080** to **088**: Rickettsioses and other arthropod-borne diseases
• **090** to **099**: Syphilis and other sexually transmitted diseases
• **100** to **104**: Other spirochetal diseases
• **110** to **118**: Mycoses
• **120** to **129**: Helminthiases
• **130** to **136**: Other infectious and parasitic diseases
• **137** to **139**: Late effects of infectious and parasitic diseases.

You'll find these abbreviations throughout the classification:
NEC = not elsewhere classified
NOS = not otherwise specified.

INTESTINAL INFECTIOUS DISEASES (001 to 009)
Excludes helminthiases (120 to 129)

001 Cholera
 001.0 Due to *Vibrio cholerae*
 001.1 Due to *Vibrio cholerae eltor*
 001.9 Cholera, unspecified

002 Typhoid and paratyphoid fevers
 002.0 Typhoid fever
  Typhoid: fever, infection, any site
 002.1 Paratyphoid fever A
 002.2 Paratyphoid fever B
 002.3 Paratyphoid fever C
 002.9 Paratyphoid fever, unspecified

003 Other salmonella infections
Includes infection or food poisoning by *Salmonella* (any serotype)
 003.0 Salmonella gastroenteritis
  salmonellosis
 003.1 Salmonella septicemia
 003.2 Localized salmonella infections
  003.20 Localized salmonella infection, unspecified
  003.21 Salmonella meningitis
  003.22 Salmonella pneumonia
  003.23 Salmonella arthritis
  003.24 Salmonella osteomyelitis
  003.29 Other
 003.8 Other specified salmonella infections
 003.9 Salmonella infection, unspecified

004 Shigellosis
Includes bacillary dysentery
 004.0 *Shigella dysenteriae*
  Infection by group A *Shigella* (Schmitz, Shiga)

004.1 *Shigella flexneri*
　Infection by group B *Shigella*
004.2 *Shigella boydii*
　Infection by group C *Shigella*
004.3 *Shigella sonnei*
　Infection by group D *Shigella*
004.8 Other specified *Shigella* infections
004.9 Shigellosis, unspecified

005 Other food poisoning (bacterial)
Excludes:
　salmonella infections (003.0 to 003.9)
　toxic effect of:
　　food contaminants (989.7)
　　noxious foodstuffs (988.0 to 988.9)
005.0 Staphylococcal food poisoning
　Staphylococcal toxemia caused by food
005.1 Botulism
　Food poisoning due to *Clostridium botuli-
　　num*
005.2 Food poisoning due to *Clostridium
　　perfringens (C. welchii)*
　Enteritis necroticans
005.3 Food poisoning due to other Clostridia
005.4 Food poisoning due to *Vibrio parahae-
　　molyticus*
005.8 Other bacterial food poisoning
　Food poisoning due to *Bacillus cereus*
　Excludes salmonella food poisoning
　　(003.0 to 003.9)
005.9 Food poisoning, unspecified

006 Amebiasis
Includes infection due to *Entamoeba histoly-
　tica*
Excludes amebiasis due to organisms other
　than *Entamoeba histolytica* (007.8)
006.0 Acute amebic dysentery without men-
　tion of abscess
　Acute amebiasis
006.1 Chronic intestinal amebiasis without
　mention of abscess
　Chronic:
　　amebiasis
　　amebic dysentery
006.2 Amebic nondysenteric colitis
006.3 Amebic liver abscess
　Hepatic amebiasis
006.4 Amebic lung abscess
　Amebic abscess of lung (and liver)
006.5 Amebic brain abscess
　Amebic abscess of brain (and liver, and
　　lung)

006.6 Amebic skin ulceration
　Cutaneous amebiasis
006.8 Amebic infection of other sites
　Amebic:
　　appendicitis
　　balanitis
　Ameboma
　Excludes specific infections by free-living
　　amebae (136.2)
006.9 Amebiasis, unspecified
　Amebiasis NOS

007 Other protozoal intestinal diseases
Includes protozoal:
　colitis
　diarrhea
　dysentery
007.0 Balantidiasis
　Infection by *Balantidium coli*
007.1 Giardiasis
　Infection by *Giardia lamblia*
　Lambliasis
007.2 Coccidiosis
　Infection by *Isospora belli* and *Isospora
　　hominis*
　Isosporiasis
007.3 Intestinal trichomoniasis
007.8 Other specified protozoal intestinal
　diseases
　Amebiasis due to organisms other than
　　Entamoeba histolytica
007.9 Unspecified protozoal intestinal dis-
　eases
　Flagellate diarrhea
　Protozoal dysentery NOS

**008 Intestinal infections due to other
　organisms**
Includes any condition classifiable to 009.0 to
　009.3 with mention of the responsible or-
　ganisms
Excludes food poisoning by these organisms
　(005.0 to 005.9)
　008.0 *Escherichia coli*
　008.1 Arizona group of paracolon bacilli
　008.2 *Aerobacter aerogenes*
　008.3 *Proteus (mirabilis) (morgani)*
　008.4 Other specified bacteria
　　008.41 *Staphylococcus*
　　　Staphylococcal enterocolitis
　　008.42 *Pseudomonas*
　　008.49 Other

008.5 Bacterial enteritis, unspecified
008.6 Enteritis due to specified virus
Enteritis due to:
adenovirus
enterovirus
008.8 Other organism NEC
Viral:
enteritis NOS
gastroenteritis
Excludes influenza with involvement of
GI tract (487.8)

009 Ill-defined intestinal infections
Excludes:
diarrheal disease or intestinal infection due
to specified organism (001.0 to 008.8)
diarrhea following GI surgery (564.4)
intestinal malabsorption (579.0 to 579.9)
ischemic enteritis (557.0 to 557.9)
other noninfectious gastroenteritis and colitis (558.1 to 558.9)
regional enteritis (555.0 to 555.9)
ulcerative colitis (556)
009.0 Infectious colitis, enteritis, and gastroenteritis
Colitis, septic
Enteritis, septic
Gastroenteritis, septic
Dysentery:
NOS
catarrhal
hemorrhagic
009.1 Colitis, enteritis, and gastroenteritis
of presumed infectious origin
Excludes:
colitis NOS (558.9)
enteritis NOS (558.9)
gastroenteritis NOS (558.9)
009.2 Infectious diarrhea
Diarrhea:
dysenteric
epidemic
Infectious diarrheal disease NOS
009.3 Diarrhea of presumed infectious origin
Excludes diarrhea NOS (558.9)

TUBERCULOSIS (010 to 018)
Includes infection by *Mycobacterium tuberculosis* (human, bovine)
Excludes:
congenital tuberculosis (771.2)
late effects of tuberculosis (137.0 to 137.4)

The following fifth-digit subclassification is
for use with categories 010 to 018:
0 = unspecified
1 = bacteriologic or histologic examination
not done
2 = bacteriologic or histologic examination
unknown (at present)
3 = tubercle bacilli found (in sputum) by microscopy
4 = tubercle bacilli not found (in sputum) by
microscopy, but found by bacterial culture
5 = tubercle bacilli not found by bacteriologic examination, but tuberculosis confirmed histologically
6 = tubercle bacilli not found by bacteriologic or histologic examination but tuberculosis confirmed by other methods (inoculation
of animals)

010 Primary tuberculous infections
010.0 Primary tuberculous complex
010.1 Tuberculous pleurisy in primary progressive tuberculosis
010.8 Other primary progressive tuberculosis
Excludes tuberculous erythema nodosum (017.1)
010.9 Primary tuberculous infection, unspecified

011 Pulmonary tuberculosis
Use additional code, if desired, to identify
any associated silicosis (502)
011.0 Tuberculosis of lung, infiltrative
011.1 Tuberculosis of lung, nodular
011.2 Tuberculosis of lung with cavitation
011.3 Tuberculosis of bronchus
Excludes isolated bronchial tuberculosis
(012.2)
011.4 Tuberculous fibrosis of lung
011.5 Tuberculous bronchiectasis
011.6 Tuberculous pneumonia (any form)
011.7 Tuberculous pneumothorax
011.8 Other specified pulmonary tuberculosis
011.9 Pulmonary tuberculosis, unspecified
Respiratory tuberculosis NOS
Tuberculosis of lung NOS

012 Other respiratory tuberculosis
Excludes respiratory tuberculosis, unspecified (011.9)
012.0 Tuberculous pleurisy
Tuberculosis of pleura

Tuberculous empyema
Tuberculous hydrothorax
Excludes:
  pleurisy with effusion without mention
    of cause (511.9)
  tuberculous pleurisy in primary pro-
    gressive tuberculosis (010.1)
012.1 Tuberculosis of intrathoracic lymph
  nodes
Tuberculosis of lymph nodes:
  hilar
  mediastinal
  tracheobronchial
Tuberculous tracheobronchial adenopathy
Excludes that specified as primary
    (010.0 to 010.9)
012.2 Isolated tracheal or bronchial tuberculosis
012.3 Tuberculous laryngitis
Tuberculosis of glottis
012.8 Other specified respiratory tuberculosis
Tuberculosis of:
  mediastinum
  nasopharynx
  nose (septum)
  sinus (any nasal)

013 Tuberculosis of meninges and CNS
  013.0 Tuberculous meningitis
  Tuberculosis of meninges (cerebral,
    spinal)
  Tuberculous leptomeningitis
  Tuberculous meningoencephalitis
  Excludes tuberculoma of meninges (013.1)
  013.1 Tuberculoma of meninges
  013.2 Tuberculoma of brain
  Tuberculosis of brain (current disease)
  013.3 Tuberculous abscess of brain
  013.4 Tuberculoma of spinal cord
  013.5 Tuberculous abscess of spinal cord
  013.6 Tuberculous encephalitis or myelitis
  013.8 Other specified tuberculosis of CNS
  013.9 Unspecified tuberculosis of CNS
  Tuberculosis of CNS NOS

**014 Tuberculosis of intestines, peritoneum, and
  mesenteric glands**
  014.0 Tuberculous peritonitis
  Tuberculous ascites
  014.8 Other
  Tuberculosis of:
    anus

intestine (large, small)
mesenteric glands
rectum
retroperitoneal (lymph nodes)
Tuberculous enteritis

015 Tuberculosis of bones and joints
Use additional code, if desired, to identify manifestation as tuberculous:
  arthropathy (711.4)
  necrosis of bone (730.8)
  osteitis (730.8)
  osteomyelitis (730.8)
  synovitis (727.01)
  tenosynovitis (727.01)
  015.0 Vertebral column
  Pott's disease
  Use additional code, if desired, to identify
    manifestation as:
    curvature of spine (Pott's, 737.4)
    kyphosis (737.4)
    spondylitis (720.81)
  015.1 Hip
  015.2 Knee
  015.5 Limb bones
  Tuberculous dactylitis
  015.6 Mastoid
  Tuberculous mastoiditis
  015.7 Other specified bone
  015.8 Other specified joint
  015.9 Tuberculosis of unspecified bones and
    joints

**016 Tuberculosis of genitourinary (GU) sys-
  tem**
  016.0 Kidney
  Renal tuberculosis
  Use additional code, if desired, to identify
    manifestation as tuberculous:
    nephropathy (583.81)
    pyelitis (590.81)
    pyelonephritis (590.81)
  016.1 Bladder
  016.2 Ureter
  016.3 Other urinary organs
  016.4 Epididymis
  016.5 Other male genital organs
  Use additional code, if desired, to identify
    manifestation as tuberculosis of:
    prostate (601.4)
    seminal vesicle (608.81)
    testis (608.81)

016.6 Tuberculous oophoritis and salpingitis
016.7 Other female genital organs
Tuberculous:
cervicitis
endometritis
016.9 GU tuberculosis, unspecified

017 Tuberculosis of other organs
017.0 Skin and subcutaneous cellular tissue
Lupus:
NOS
exedens
vulgaris
Scrofuloderma
Tuberculosis:
colliquativa
cutis
lichenoides
papulonecrotica
verrucosa cutis
Excludes:
lupus erythematosus (695.4)
disseminated (710.0)
017.1 Erythema nodosum with hypersensitivity reaction in tuberculosis
Bazin's disease
Erythema:
induratum
nodosum, tuberculous
Tuberculosis indurativa
Excludes erythema nodosum NOS
(695.2)
017.2 Peripheral lymph nodes
Scofula
Scrofulous abscess
Tuberculous adenitis
Excludes:
tuberculosis of lymph nodes
bronchial and mediastinal (012.1)
mesenteric and retroperitoneal (014.8)
tuberculous tracheobronchial adenopathy (012.1)
017.3 Eye
Use additional code, if desired, to identify manifestation as tuberculous:
chorioretinitis, disseminated (363.13)
episcleritis (379.09)
interstitial keratitis (370.59)
iridocyclitis, chronic (364.11)
keratoconjunctivitis (phlyctenular)
(370.31)
017.4 Ear
Tuberculosis of ear

Tuberculous otitis media
Excludes tuberculous mastoiditis (015.6)
017.5 Thyroid gland
017.6 Adrenal glands
Addison's disease, tuberculous
017.7 Spleen
017.8 Esophagus
017.9 Other specified organs
Use additional code, if desired, to identify manifestation as tuberculosis of:
endocardium (any valve, 424.91)
myocardium (422.0)
pericardium (420.0)

018 Miliary tuberculosis
Includes tuberculosis:
disseminated
generalized
miliary, whether of a single specified site, multiple sites, or unspecified site
polyserositis
018.0 Acute miliary tuberculosis
018.8 Other specified miliary tuberculosis
018.9 Miliary tuberculosis, unspecified

ZOONOTIC BACTERIAL DISEASES (020 to 027)

020 Plague
Includes infection by *Yersinia (Pasteurella) pestis*
020.0 Bubonic
020.1 Cellulocutaneous
020.2 Septicemic
020.3 Primary pneumonic
020.4 Secondary pneumonic
020.5 Pneumonic, unspecified
020.8 Other specified types of plague
Abortive plague
Ambulatory plague
Pestis minor
020.9 Plague, unspecified

021 Tularemia
Includes:
deerfly fever
infection by *Francisella (Pasteurella) tularensis*
rabbit fever
021.0 Ulceroglandular tularemia
021.1 Enteric tularemia
Tularemia:
cryptogenic

intestinal
typhoidal
021.2 Pulmonary tularemia
Bronchopneumonic tularemia
021.3 Oculoglandular tularemia
021.8 Other specified tularemia
Tularemia:
generalized or disseminated
glandular
021.9 Unspecified tularemia

022 Anthrax
022.0 Cutaneous anthrax
Malignant pustule
022.1 Pulmonary anthrax
Respiratory anthrax
Wool-sorters' disease
022.2 GI anthrax
022.3 Anthrax septicemia
022.8 Other specified manifestations of anthrax
022.9 Anthrax, unspecified

023 Brucellosis
Includes:
fever:
Malta
Mediterranean
undulant
023.0 *Brucella melitensis*
023.1 *Brucella abortus*
023.2 *Brucella suis*
023.3 *Brucella canis*
023.8 Other brucellosis
Infection by more than one organism
023.9 Brucellosis, unspecified

024 Glanders
Infection by:
Actinobacillus mallei
Malleomyces mallei
Pseudomonas mallei
Farcy
Malleus

025 Melioidosis
Infection by:
Malleomyces pseudomallei
Pseudomonas pseudomallei
Whitmore's bacillus
Pseudoglanders

026 Rat-bite fever
026.0 Spirillary fever
Rat-bite fever due to *Spirillum minor*
Sodoku
026.1 Streptobacillary fever
Epidemic arthritic erythema
Haverhill fever
Rat-bite fever due to *Streptobacillus moniliformis*
026.9 Unspecified rat-bite fever

027 Other zoonotic bacterial diseases
027.0 Listeriosis
Infection by *Listeria monocytogenes*
Septicemia by *Listeria monocytogenes*
Use additional code, if desired, to identify manifestation as meningitis (320.7)
Excludes congenital listeriosis (771.2)
027.1 *Erysipelothrix* infection
Erysipeloid (of Rosenbach)
Infection by *Erysipelothrix insidiosa (E. rhusiopathiae)*
Septicemia by *Erysipelothrix insidiosa (E. rhusiopathiae)*
027.2 Pasteurellosis
Pasteurella pseudotuberculosis infection
Mesenteric adenitis by *Pasteurella multocida (P. septica)*
Septic infection (cat or dog bite) by *Pasteurella multocida (P. septica)*
Excludes infection by:
Francisella (Pasteurella) tularensis (021.0 to 021.9)
Yersinia (Pasteurella) pestis (020.0 to 020.9)
027.8 Other specified zoonotic bacterial diseases
027.9 Zoonotic bacterial disease, unspecified

OTHER BACTERIAL DISEASES (030 to 041)
Excludes:
bacterial venereal diseases (098.0 to 099.9)
bartonellosis (088.0)

030 Leprosy
Includes:
Hansen's disease
infection by *Mycobacterium leprae*

030.0 Lepromatous (type L)
Lepromatous leprosy (macular, diffuse, infiltrated, nodular, neuritic)
030.1 Tuberculoid (type T)
Tuberculoid leprosy (mascular) (maculoanesthetic, major, minor, neuritic)
030.2 Indeterminate (group I)
Indeterminate (uncharacteristic) leprosy (macular, neuritic)
030.3 Borderline (group B)
Borderline or dimorphous leprosy (infiltrated, neuritic)
030.8 Other specified leprosy
030.9 Leprosy, unspecified

031 Diseases due to other mycobacteria
031.0 Pulmonary
Battey disease
Infection by *Mycobacterium:*
  avium
  intracellulare
  kansasii
031.1 Cutaneous
Buruli ulcer
Infection by *Mycobacterium:*
  marinum (M. balnei)
  ulcerans
031.8 Other specified mycobacterial diseases
031.9 Unspecified diseases due to mycobacteria
Atypical mycobacterium infection NOS

032 Diphtheria
Includes infection by *Corynebacterium diphtheriae*
032.0 Faucial diphtheria
Membranous angina, diphtheritic
032.1 Nasopharyngeal diphtheria
032.2 Anterior nasal diphtheria
032.3 Laryngeal diphtheria
Laryngotracheitis, diphtheritic
032.8 Other specified diphtheria
  032.81 Conjunctival diphtheria
  Pseudomembranous diphtheritic conjunctivitis
  032.82 Diphtheritic myocarditis
  032.83 Diphtheritic peritonitis
  032.84 Diphtheritic cystitis
  032.85 Cutaneous diphtheria
  032.89 Other
032.9 Diphtheria, unspecified

033 Whooping cough
Includes pertussis
Use additional code, if desired, to identify any associated pneumonia (484.3)
033.0 *Bordetella pertussis*
033.1 *Bordetella parapertussis*
033.8 Whooping cough due to other specified organism
Bordetella bronchiseptica
033.9 Whooping cough, unspecified organism

034 Streptococcal sore throat and scarlet fever
034.0 Streptococcal sore throat
Septic:
  angina
  sore throat
Streptococcal:
  angina
  laryngitis
  pharyngitis
  tonsillitis
034.1 Scarlet fever
Scarlatina
Excludes parascarlatina (057.8)

035 Erysipelas
Excludes postpartum or puerperal erysipelas (670)

036 Meningococcal infection
036.0 Meningococcal meningitis
Cerebrospinal fever (meningococcal)
Meningitis:
  cerebrospinal
  epidemic
036.1 Meningococcal encephalitis
036.2 Meningococcemia
Meningococcal septicemia
036.3 Waterhouse-Friderichsen syndrome, meningococcal
Meningococcal hemorrhagic adrenalitis
Meningococcic adrenal syndrome
Waterhouse-Friderichsen syndrome NOS
036.4 Meningococcal carditis
  036.40 Meningococcal carditis, unspecified
  036.41 Meningococcal pericarditis
  036.42 Meningococcal endocarditis
  036.43 Meningococcal myocarditis
036.8 Other specified meningococcal infections

036.81 Meningococcal optic neuritis
036.82 Meningococcal arthropathy
036.89 Other
036.9 Meningococcal infection, unspecified
Meningococcal infection NOS

037 Tetanus
Excludes tetanus:
 complicating:
  abortion (634 to 638 with .0, 639.0)
  ectopic or molar pregnancy (639.0)
 neonatorum (771.3)
 puerperal (670)

038 Septicemia
Excludes:
 during labor (659.3)
 following ectopic or molar pregnancy
  (639.0)
 following infusion, injection, transfusion, or
  vaccination (999.3)
 postoperative (998.5)
 postpartum, puerperal (670)
 that complicates abortion (634 to 638 with
  .0, 639.0)
038.0 Streptococcal septicemia
038.1 Staphylococcal septicemia
038.2 Pneumococcal septicemia
038.3 Septicemia due to anaerobes
 Septicemia due to bacteroides
 Excludes:
  gas gangrene (040.0)
  infection due to anaerobic streptococci (038.0)
038.4 Septicemia due to other gram-negative organisms
 038.40 Gram-negative organism, unspecified
 Gram-negative septicemia NOS
 038.41 *Haemophilus influenzae*
 038.42 *Escherichia coli*
 038.43 *Pseudomonas*
 038.44 *Serratia*
 038.49 Other
038.8 Other specified septicemias
 Excludes:
  septicemia due to:
   anthrax (022.3)
   gonococcal (098.89)
   herpetic (054.5)
   meningococcal (036.2)
  septicemic plague (020.2)

038.9 Septicemia, unspecified
 Septicemia NOS
 Excludes bacteremia NOS (790.7)

039 Actinomycotic infections
Includes:
 actinomycotic mycetoma
 infection by Actinomycetales, such as species of *Actinomyces, Actinomadura,
  Nocardia, Streptomyces*
 actinomycotic maduromyucosis
 actinomycotic schizomycetoma
039.0 Cutaneous
 Erythrasma
 Trichomycosis axillaris
039.1 Pulmonary
 Thoracic actinomycosis
039.2 Abdominal
039.3 Cervicofacial
039.4 Madura foot
 Excludes Madura foot due to mycotic infection (117.4)
039.8 Of other specified sites
039.9 Of unspecified site
 Actinomycosis NOS
 Maduromycosis NOS
 Nocardiosis NOS

040 Other bacterial diseases
Excludes:
 bacteremia NOS (790.7)
 bacterial infection NOS (041.9)
040.0 Gas gangrene
 Gas bacillus infection
  or gangrene
 Infection by *Clostridium:*
  histolyticum
  oedematiens
  perfringens (welchii)
  septicum
  sordellii
 Malignant edema
 Myonecrosis, clostridial
 Myositis, clostridial
040.1 Rhinoscleroma
040.2 Whipple's disease
 Intestinal lipodystrophy
040.3 Necrobacillosis
040.8 Other specified bacterial diseases
 040.81 Tropical pyomyositis
 040.89 Other

**041 Bacterial infection in conditions classi-
fied elsewhere and of unspecified site**

Note: This category is provided to be used
as an additional code where it is desired
to identify the bacterial agent in diseases classified elsewhere. This category will also be used to classify
bacterial infections of unspecified nature
or site.

Excludes:
  bacteremia NOS (790.7)
  septicemia (038.0 to 038.9)
  041.0 Streptococcus
  041.1 Staphylococcus
  041.2 Pneumococcus
  041.3 Friedländer's bacillus
  Infection by *Klebsiella pneumoniae*
  041.4 *Escherichia coli*
  041.5 *Haemophilus influenzae*
  041.6 *Proteus (mirabilis, morganii)*
  041.7 *Pseudomonas*
  041.8 Other specified bacterial infections
  Aerobacter aerogenes
  Eaton's agent
  Mima polymorpha
  Mycoplasma
  Pleuropneumonia-like organisms
  Serratia
  Other cocci NEC
  041.9 Bacterial infection, unspecified

**HUMAN IMMUNODEFICIENCY VIRUS (HIV)
INFECTION (042 to 044)**

**042 Human immunodeficiency virus infection
with specified conditions**

Includes acquired immunodeficiency syndrome (AIDS)
  042.0 With specified infections
  Includes only the following with HIV infection:
    candidiasis of lung (112.4)
    coccidiosis (007.2)
      cryptosporidiosis (007.2)
      isosporiasis (007.2)
    cryptococcosis (117.5)
    pneumocystosis (136.3)
    progressive multifocal, leukoencepha-
lopathy (046.3)
    toxoplasmosis (130)
  042.1 Causing other specified infections
  Includes only the following due to HIV infection:
    candidiasis

acute or subacute endocarditis (421.0,
  421.9)
acute or subacute myocarditis (422.90
  to 422.99)
  disseminated (112.5)
  of:
    mouth (112.0)
    skin and nails (112.3)
    other and unspecified sites (112.8,
      112.9; excludes 112.1, 112.2,
      112.4)
coccidioidomycosis (114)
cytomegalic inclusion disease (078.5)
herpes simplex (054)
herpes zoster (053)
histoplasmosis (115)
microsporidiosis (136.8)
other and unspecified myobacteriosis
  (031.8, 031.9; excludes 031.0,
  031.1)
Nocardia infection (039)
opportunistic mycoses (118)
pneumonia:
  NOS (486)
  other bacterial pneumonia (482.0 to
    482.9)
  pneumococcal (481)
  viral NEC and NOS (480.0, 480.9)
Salmonella infections (003.1 to 003.9;
  excludes gastroenteritis [003.9])
septicemia (038)
strongyloidiasis (127.2)
tuberculosis (010 to 018)
042.2 With specified malignant neoplasms
Includes only the following with HIV infection:
  Burkitt's tumor or lymphoma (200.2)
  Kaposi's sarcoma (176.0 to 176.9)
  lymphoma:
    histiocytic (200.0)
    large cell (200.0)
  immunoblastic sarcoma (200.8)
  primary lymphoma of the brain (202.8)
  reticulosarcoma (200.0)
042.9 AIDS, unspecified
AIDS with other conditions classifiable
  elsewhere except as in 042.0 to
  042.2

**043 HIV infection causing other specified
conditions**

Includes:
  AIDS-like syndrome
  AIDS-related complex (ARC)
Excludes HIV infection classifiable to 042

043.0 Causing lymphadenopathy
  Enlarged lymph nodes due to HIV infection (785.6)
  Swollen glands due to HIV infection (785.6)
043.1 Causing specified diseases of the CNS
  Includes only the following due to HIV infection:
  CNS:
    demyelinating disease NOS (341.9)
    disorders NOS (348.9, 349.9)
    other and unspecified nonarthropod-borne viral diseases (049.8, 049.9)
    other and unspecified slow virus infection (046.8, 046.9)
  dementia:
    NOS (298.9)
    organic (294.9)
    presenile (290.1)
    encephalitis (323.8, 323.9)
    encephalomyelitis (323.8, 323.9)
    encephalopathy (348.3)
    myelitis (323.8, 323.9)
    myelopathy (336.9)
    organic brain syndrome NOS (nonpsychotic, 310.9; psychotic, 294.9)
043.2 Causing other disorders involving the immune mechanism
043.3 Causing other specified conditions
  Includes only the following due to HIV infection:
    abnormal weight loss (783.2)
    abnormality, respiratory (786.0)
    agranulocytosis (288.0)
    anemia:
      NOS (285.9)
      other and unspecified aplastic (284.8, 284.9)
      deficiency (280 to 281)
      acquired hemolytic (283)
    arthritis:
      pyogenic (711.0)
      infective (711.9)
    blindness or low vision (369)
    unspecified blood and blood-forming organs disease (289.9)
    cachexia (799.4)
    dermatomycosis (111)
    dermatophytosis (110)
    diarrhea (noninfectious, 558)
      infectious (009)

disease or disorder NOS:
  blood and blood-forming organs (289.9)
  salivary gland (527.9)
  skin and subcutaneous tissue (709.9)
dyspnea (786.0)
fatigue (780.7)
fever (780.6)
gastroenteritis (noninfectious, 558)
  infectious (009)
hepatomegaly (789.1)
hyperhidrosis (780.8)
hypersplenism (289.4)
infection: intestinal, ill-defined (009)
lack of expected physiological development in infant (783.4)
leukoplakia of oral mucosa (tongue) (528.6)
malabsorption, intestinal (579.9)
malaise (780.7)
nephritis and nephropathy (580 to 583)
neuralgia NOS (729.2)
neuritis NOS (729.2)
nutritional deficiencies (260 to 269)
pneumonitis, lymphoid, interstitial (516.8)
polyneuropathy (357.0, 357.8, 357.9)
pyrexia (780.6)
radiculitis NOS (729.2)
rash NOS (782.1)
retinal vascular changes (362.1)
retinopathy, background (362.1)
secondary cardiomyopathy (425.9)
splenomegaly (789.2)
thrombocytopenia, secondary and unspecified (287.4, 287.5)
volume depletion (276.5)
043.9 ARC, unspecified
ARC with other conditions classifiable elsewhere except as in 042.0 to 043.3

044 Other HIV infection
Excludes HIV infection classifiable to 042 or 043
044.0 Causing specified acute infections
  Includes only the following due to HIV infection:
    acute lymphadenitis (683)
    aseptic meningitis (047.9)
    viral infection ("infectious mononucleosis-like syndrome," 079.9)

044.9 HIV infection, unspecified
HIV infection with other conditions classifiable elsewhere except as in 042.0 to 044.0

POLIOMYELITIS AND OTHER NONARTHROPOD-BORNE VIRAL DISEASES OF THE CNS (045 to 049)

045 Acute poliomyelitis
Excludes late effects of acute poliomyelitis (138)

The following fifth-digit subclassification is for use with category 045:
0 = poliovirus, unspecified type
1 = poliovirus type I
2 = poliovirus type II
3 = poliovirus type III

045.0 Acute paralytic poliomyelitis
Infantile paralysis (acute, specified as bulbar)
Poliomyelitis (acute, anterior, specified as bulbar)
Polioencephalitis (acute, bulbar)
Polioencephalomyelitis (acute, anterior, bulbar) specified as bulbar

045.1 Acute poliomyelitis with other paralysis
Paralysis:
acute atrophic, spinal
infantile, paralytic
Poliomyelitis (acute, with paralysis except bulbar):
anterior
epidemic

045.2 Acute nonparalytic poliomyelitis
Poliomyelitis (acute, specified as nonparalytic):
anterior
epidemic

045.9 Acute poliomyelitis, unspecified
Infantile paralysis (unspecified whether paralytic or nonparalytic)
Poliomyelitis (acute, unspecified whether paralytic or nonparalytic):
anterior
epidemic

046 Slow viral infection of CNS
046.0 Kuru
046.1 Jakob-Creutzfeldt disease
Subacute spongiform encephalopathy

046.2 Subacute sclerosing panencephalitis
Dawson's inclusion body encephalitis
van Bogaert's sclerosing leukoencephalitis

046.3 Progressive multifocal leukoencephalopathy
Multifocal leukoencephalopathy NOS

046.8 Other specified slow viral infection of the CNS

046.9 Unspecified slow virus infection of the CNS

047 Meningitis due to enterovirus
Includes meningitis:
abacterial
aseptic
viral
Excludes meningitis due to:
adenovirus (049.1)
arthropod-borne virus (060.0 to 066.9)
leptospira (100.81)
virus of:
herpes simplex (054.72)
herpes zoster (053.0)
lymphocytic choriomeningitis (049.0)
mumps (072.1)
poliomyelitis (045.0 to 045.9)
any other infection specifically classified elsewhere

047.0 Coxsackievirus
047.1 ECHO virus
Meningo-eruptive syndrome
047.8 Other specified viral meningitis
047.9 Unspecified viral meningitis
Viral meningitis NOS

048 Other enterovirus diseases of the CNS
Boston exanthem

049 Other nonarthropod-borne viral diseases of the CNS
Excludes late effects of viral encephalitis (139.0)

049.0 Lymphocytic choriomeningitis
Lymphocytic:
meningitis (serous, benign)
meningoencephalitis (serous, benign)
049.1 Meningitis due to adenovirus
049.8 Other specified nonarthropod-borne viral diseases of the CNS
Encephalitis:
acute:
inclusion body

necrotizing
epidemic
lethargica
Rio Bravo
von Economo's disease
049.9 Unspecified nonarthropod-borne
viral diseases of the CNS
Viral encephalitis NOS

**VIRAL DISEASES ACCOMPANIED BY EXAN-
THEM (050 to 057)**
Excludes:
anthropod-borne viral diseases (060.0 to
066.9)
Boston exanthem (048)

050 Smallpox
050.0 Variola major
Hemorrhagic (pustular) smallpox
Malignant smallpox
Purpura variolosa
050.1 Alastrim
Variola minor
050.2 Modified smallpox
Varioloid
050.9 Smallpox, unspecified

051 Cowpox and paravaccinia
051.0 Cowpox
Vaccinia not from vaccination
Excludes vaccinia (generalized, from
vaccination, 999.0)
051.1 Pseudocowpox
Milkers' node
051.2 Contagious pustular dermatitis
Ecthyma contagiosum
Orf
051.9 Paravaccinia, unspecified

052 Chickenpox
052.0 Postvaricella encephalitis
Postchickenpox encephalitis
052.1 Varicella (hemorrhagic) pneumonitis
052.7 With other specified complications
052.8 With unspecified complications
052.9 Varicella without mention of complication
Chickenpox NOS
Varicella NOS

053 Herpes zoster
Includes:

shingles
zona
053.0 With meningitis
053.1 With other nervous system complications
053.10 With unspecified nervous system
complications
053.11 Geniculate herpes zoster
Herpetic geniculate ganglionitis
053.12 Postherpetic trigeminal neuralgia
053.13 Postherpetic polyneuropathy
053.19 Other
053.2 With ophthalmic complications
053.20 Herpes zoster dermatitis of eyelid
Herpes zoster ophthalmicus
053.21 Herpes zoster keratoconjunctivitis
053.22 Herpes zoster iridocyclitis
053.29 Other
053.7 With other specified complications
053.71 Otitis externa due to herpes zoster
053.79 Other
053.8 With unspecified complications
053.9 Herpes zoster without mention of
complications
Herpes zoster NOS

054 Herpes simplex
Excludes congenital herpes simplex (771.2)
054.0 Eczema herpeticum
Kaposi's varicelliform eruption
054.1 Genital herpes
054.10 Genital herpes, unspecified
Herpes progenitalis
054.11 Herpetic vulvovaginitis
054.12 Herpetic ulceration of vulva
054.13 Herpetic infection of penis
054.19 Other
054.2 Herpetic gingivostomatitis
054.3 Herpetic meningoencephalitis
Herpes encephalitis
Simian B disease
054.4 With ophthalmic complications
054.40 With unspecified ophthalmic
complications
054.41 Herpes simplex dermatitis of eyelid
054.42 Dendritic keratitis
054.43 Herpes simplex disciform keratitis

054.44 Herpes simplex iridocyclitis
054.49 Other
054.5 Herpetic septicemia
054.6 Herpetic whitlow
    Herpetic felon
054.7 With other specified complications
    054.71 Visceral herpes simplex
    054.72 Herpes simplex meningitis
    054.73 Herpes simplex otitis externa
    054.79 Other
054.8 With unspecified complications
054.9 Herpes simplex without mention of
    complications

055 Measles
Includes:
    morbilli
    rubeola
055.0 Postmeasles encephalitis
055.1 Postmeasles pneumonia
055.2 Postmeasles otitis media
055.7 With other specified complications
    055.71 Measles keratoconjunctivitis
    Measles keratitis
    055.79 Other
055.8 With unspecified complications
055.9 Measles without mention of compli-
    cations

056 Rubella
Includes German measles
Excludes congenital rubella (771.0)
    056.0 With neurologic complications
        056.00 With unspecified neurologic
        complications
        056.01 Encephalomyelitis due to rubella
        Encephalitis due to rubella
        Meningoencephalitis due to rubella
        056.09 Other
    056.7 With other specified complications
        056.71 Arthritis due to rubella
        056.79 Other
    056.8 With unspecified complications
    056.9 Rubella without mention of compli-
        cations

057 Other viral exanthemata
    057.0 Erythema infectiosum (fifth disease)
    057.8 Other specified viral exanthemata
    Dukes (Filatov-Dukes') disease
    Exanthema subitum (sixth disease)
    Fourth disease
    Parascarlatina

    Pseudoscarlatina
    Roseola infantum
    057.9 Viral exanthem, unspecified

**ARTHROPOD-BORNE VIRAL DISEASES
(060 to 066)**
Use additional code, if desired, to identify
    any associated meningitis (321.2)
Excludes late effects of viral encephalitis
    (139.0)

060 Yellow fever
    060.0 Sylvatic
    Yellow fever:
        jungle
        sylvan
    060.1 Urban
    060.9 Yellow fever, unspecified

061 Dengue
    Breakbone fever
    Excludes hemorrhagic fever caused by
        dengue virus (065.4)

062 Mosquito-borne viral encephalitis
    062.0 Japanese encephalitis
    Japanese B encephalitis
    062.1 Western equine encephalitis
    062.2 Eastern equine encephalitis
    Excludes Venezuelan equine encephali-
        tis (066.2)
    062.3 St. Louis encephalitis
    062.4 Australian encephalitis
    Australian arboencephalitis
    Australian X disease
    Murray Valley encephalitis
    062.5 California virus encephalitis
    Encephalitis:
        California
        La Crosse
    Tahyna fever
    062.8 Other specified mosquito-borne viral
        encephalitis
    Encephalitis by Ilheus virus
    062.9 Mosquito-borne viral encephalitis,
        unspecified

063 Tick-borne viral encephalitis
Includes diphasic meningoencephalitis
    063.0 Russian spring-summer (taiga) en-
        cephalitis
    063.1 Louping ill

063.2 Central European encephalitis
063.8 Other specified tick-borne encephalitis
Langat encephalitis
Powassan encephalitis
063.9 Tick-borne viral encephalitis, unspecified

064 Viral encephalitis transmitted by other and unspecified arthropods
Arthropod-borne viral encephalitis, vector unknown
Negishi virus encephalitis
Excludes viral encephalitis NOS (049.9)

065 Arthropod-borne hemorrhagic fever
065.0 Crimean hemorrhagic fever (CHF Congo virus)
Central Asian hemorrhagic fever
065.1 Omsk hemorrhagic fever
065.2 Kyasanur Forest disease
065.3 Other tick-borne hemorrhagic fever
065.4 Mosquito-borne hemorrhagic fever
Chikungunya hemorrhagic fever
Dengue hemorrhagic fever
Excludes:
Chikungunya fever (066.3)
dengue (061)
yellow fever (060.0 to 060.9)
065.8 Other specified arthropod-borne hemorrhagic fever
Mite-borne hemorrhagic fever
065.9 Arthropod-borne hemorrhagic fever, unspecified
Arbovirus hemorrhagic fever NOS

066 Other arthropod-borne viral diseases
066.0 Phlebotomus fever
Changuinola fever
Sandfly fever
066.1 Tick-borne fever
Nairobi sheep disease
Tick fever:
American
mountain
Colorado
Kemerovo
Quaranfil
066.2 Venezuelan equine fever
Venezuelan equine encephalitis
066.3 Other mosquito-borne fevers
Fever (viral):
Bunyamwera

Bwamba
Chikungunya
Guama
Mayaro
Mucambo
O'nyong-nyong
Oropouche
Pixuna
Rift valley
Ross river
Wesselsbron
West Nile
Zika
Excludes:
dengue (061)
yellow fever (060.0 to 060.9)
066.8 Other specified arthropod-borne viral diseases
Chandipura fever
Piry fever
066.9 Arthropod-borne viral disease, unspecified
Arbovirus infection NOS

OTHER DISEASES DUE TO VIRUSES AND CHLAMYDIAE (070 to 079)

070 Viral hepatitis
Excludes cytomegalic inclusion virus hepatitis (078.5)
070.0 Viral hepatitis A with hepatic coma
070.1 Viral hepatitis A without mention of hepatic coma
Infectious hepatitis
070.2 Viral hepatitis B with hepatic coma
The following fifth-digit subclassification is for use with the category 070.2:
0 = without mention of hepatitis delta
1 = with hepatitis delta
070.3 Viral hepatitis B without mention of hepatic coma
Serum hepatitis
The following fifth-digit subclassification is for use with the category 070.3:
0 = without mention of hepatitis delta
1 = with hepatitis delta
070.4 Other specified viral hepatitis with hepatic coma
The following fifth-digit subclassification is for use with the category 070.4:

1 = Hepatitis C
2 = Hepatitis delta without mention of active hepatitis B disease
Hepatitis delta with hepatitis B carrier state
3 = Hepatitis E
9 = Other specified viral hepatitis
070.5 Other specified viral hepatitis without mention of hepatic coma
The following fifth-digit subclassification is for use with the category 070.5:
1 = Hepatitis C
2 = Hepatitis delta without mention of active hepatitis B disease
Hepatitis delta with hepatitis B carrier state
3 = Hepatitis E
9 = Other specified viral hepatitis
070.6 Unspecified viral hepatitis with hepatic coma
070.9 Unspecified viral hepatitis without mention of hepatic coma
Viral hepatitis NOS

071 Rabies
Hydrophobia
Lyssa

072 Mumps
072.0 Mumps orchitis
072.1 Mumps meningitis
072.2 Mumps encephalitis
Mumps meningoencephalitis
072.3 Mumps pancreatitis
072.7 Mumps with other specified complications
072.71 Mumps hepatitis
072.72 Mumps polyneuropathy
072.79 Other
072.8 Mumps with unspecified complications
072.9 Mumps without mention of complications
Epidemic parotitis
Infectious parotitis

073 Ornithosis
Includes:
parrot fever
psittacosis
073.0 With pneumonia
Lobular pneumonitis due to ornithosis
073.7 With other specified complications

073.8 With unspecified complications
073.9 Ornithosis, unspecified

074 Specific diseases due to Coxsackie virus
Excludes:
Coxsackie virus:
infection NOS (079.2)
meningitis (047.0)
074.0 Herpangina
Vesicular pharyngitis
074.1 Epidemic pleurodynia
Bornholm disease
Devil's grip
Epidemic:
myalgia
myositis
074.2 Coxsackie carditis
074.20 Coxsackie carditis, unspecified
074.21 Coxsackie pericarditis
074.22 Coxsackie endocarditis
074.23 Coxsackie myocarditis
Aseptic myocarditis of newborn
074.3 Hand, foot, and mouth disease
Vesicular stomatitis and exanthem
074.8 Other specified diseases due to coxsackie virus
Acute lymphonodular pharyngitis

075 Infectious mononucleosis
Glandular fever
Monocytic angina
Pfeiffer's disease

076 Trachoma
Excludes late effect of trachoma (139.1)
076.0 Initial stage
Trachoma dubium
076.1 Active stage
Granular conjunctivitis (trachomatous)
Trachomatous
follicular conjunctivitis
pannus
076.9 Trachoma, unspecified
Trachoma NOS

077 Other diseases of conjunctiva due to viruses and Chlamydiae
Excludes ophthalmic complications of viral diseases classified elsewhere
077.0 Inclusion conjunctivitis
Paratrachoma
Swimming pool conjunctivitis

Excludes inclusion blennorrhea (neonatal, 771.6)

077.1 Epidemic keratoconjunctivitis
Shipyard eye

077.2 Pharyngoconjunctival fever
Viral pharyngoconjunctivitis

077.3 Other adenoviral conjunctivitis
Acute adenoviral follicular conjunctivitis

077.4 Epidemic hemorrhagic conjunctivitis
Apollo:
conjunctivitis
disease
Conjunctivitis due to enterovirus type 70
Hemorrhagic conjunctivitis (acute, epidemic)

077.8 Other viral conjunctivitis
Newcastle conjunctivitis

077.9 Unspecified diseases of conjunctiva due to viruses and Chlamydiae
Viral conjunctivitis NOS

078 Other diseases due to viruses and Chlamydiae
Excludes:
viral infection NOS (079.0 to 079.9)
viremia NOS (790.8)

078.0 Molluscum contagiosum

078.1 Viral warts
Condyloma acuminatum
Verruca (vulgaris, plana, plantaris)
Warts (infectious)

078.2 Sweating fever
Miliary fever
Sweating disease

078.3 Cat-scratch disease
Benign lymphoreticulosis (of inoculation)
Cat-scratch fever

078.4 Foot-and-mouth disease
Aphthous fever
Epizootic:
aphthae
stomatitis

078.5 Cytomegalic inclusion disease
Salivary gland virus disease
Use additional code, if desired, to identify manifestation as:
cytomegalic inclusion virus:
hepatitis (573.1)
pneumonia (484.1)
Excludes congenital cytomegalovirus infection (771.1)

078.6 Hemorrhagic nephrosonephritis
Hemorrhagic fever:

epidemic
Korean
Russian
with renal syndrome

078.7 Arenaviral hemorrhagic fever
Hemorrhagic fever:
Argentinian
Bolivian
Junin virus
Machupo virus

078.8 Other specified diseases due to viruses and Chlamydiae
Excludes:
epidemic diarrhea (009.2)
lymphogranuloma venereum (099.1)

078.81 Epidemic vertigo

078.82 Epidemic vomiting syndrome
Winter vomiting disease

078.89 Other
Epidemic cervical myalgia
Marburg disease
Tanapox

079 Viral infection in conditions classified elsewhere and of unspecified site
Note: This category is provided to be used as an additional code where it is desired to identify the viral agent in diseases classifiable elsewhere. This category will also be used to classify virus infection of unspecified nature or site.

079.0 Adenovirus

079.1 ECHO virus

079.2 Coxsackie virus

079.3 Rhinovirus

079.8 Other specified viral infections

079.9 Unspecified viral infection
Viral infection NOS
Excludes viremia NOS (790.8)

RICKETTSIOSES AND OTHER ARTHROPOD-BORNE DISEASES (080 to 088)
Excludes arthropod-borne viral diseases (060.0 to 066.9)

080 Louse-borne (epidemic) typhus
Typhus (fever):
classic
epidemic
exanthematic NOS
louse-borne

081 Other typhus
  081.0 Murine (endemic) typhus
    Typhus (fever):
      endemic
      flea-borne
  081.1 Brill's disease
    Brill-Zinsser disease
    Recrudescent typhus (fever)
  081.2 Scrub typhus
    Japanese river fever
    Kedani fever
    Mite-borne typhus
    Tsutsugamushi
  081.9 Typhus, unspecified
    Typhus (fever) NOS

082 Tick-borne rickettsioses
  082.0 Spotted fevers
    Rocky Mountain spotted fever
    São Paulo fever
  082.1 Boutonneuse fever
    African tick typhus
    India tick typhus
    Kenya tick typhus
    Marseilles fever
    Mediterranean tick fever
  082.2 North Asian tick fever
    Siberian tick typhus
  082.3 Queensland tick typhus
  082.8 Other specified tick-borne rickett-
    sioses
    Lone Star fever
  082.9 Tick-borne rickettsiosis, unspecified
    Tick-borne typhus NOS

083 Other rickettsioses
  083.0 Q fever
  083.1 Trench fever
    Quintan fever
    Wolhynian fever
  083.2 Rickettsial pox
    Vesicular rickettsiosis
  083.8 Other specified rickettsioses
  083.9 Rickettsiosis, unspecified

084 Malaria
Note: Subcategories 084.0 to 084.6 exclude
  the listed conditions with mention of pernicious complications (084.8 to 084.9).
Excludes congenital malaria (771.2)
  084.0 Falciparum malaria (malignant ter-
    tian)
    Malaria (fever):

      by *Plasmodium falciparum*
      subtertian
  084.1 Vivax malaria (benign tertian)
    Malaria (fever) by *Plasmodium vivax*
  084.2 Quartan malaria
    Malaria (fever) by *Plasmodium malariae*
    Malariae malaria
  084.3 Ovale malaria
    Malaria (fever) by *Plasmodium ovale*
  084.4 Other malaria
    Monkey malaria
  084.5 Mixed malaria
    Malaria (fever) by more than one para-
    site
  084.6 Malaria, unspecified
    Malaria (fever) NOS
  084.7 Induced malaria
    Therapeutically induced malaria
    Excludes:
      accidental infection from syringe
      blood transfusion, etc. (084.0 to 084.6
        above, according to parasite spe-
        cies)
      transmission from mother to child dur-
        ing delivery (771.2)
  084.8 Blackwater fever
    Hemoglobinuric:
      fever (bilious)
      malaria
    Malarial hemoglobinuria
  084.9 Other pernicious complications of
    malaria
    Algid malaria
    Cerebral malaria
    Use additional code, if desired, to iden-
      tify complication as:
    malarial:
      hepatitis (573.2)
      nephrosis (581.81)

085 Leishmaniasis
  085.0 Visceral (Kala-azar)
    Dumdum fever
    Infection by *Leishmania:*
      donovani
      infantum
    Leishmaniasis:
      dermal
      post-kala-azar
      Mediterranean
      visceral (Indian)
  085.1 Cutaneous, urban
    Aleppo boil

Baghdad boil
Delhi boil
Infection by:
 Leishmania tropica (minor)
Leishmaniasis, cutaneous:
 dry form
 late
 recurrent
 ulcerating
 Oriental sore
085.2 Cutaneous, Asian desert
Infection by *Leishmania tropica major*
Leishmaniasis, cutaneous:
 acute necrotizing
 rural
 wet form
 zoonotic form
085.3 Cutaneous, Ethiopian
Infection by *Leishmania ethiopica*
Leishmaniasis, cutaneous:
 diffuse
 lepromatous
085.4 Cutaneous, American
Chiclero ulcer
Infection by *Leishmania mexicana*
Leishmaniasis tegmentaria diffusa
085.5 Mucocutaneous (American)
Espundia
Infection by *Leishmania braziliensis*
Uta
085.9 Leishmaniasis, unspecified

086 Trypanosomiasis
Use additional code, if desired, to identify
 manifestations as:
trypanosomiasis:
 encephalitis (323.2)
 meningitis (321.3)
086.0 Chagas' disease with heart involvement
American trypanosomiasis
Infection by *Trypanosoma cruzi*
Any condition classifiable to 086.2
086.1 Chagas' disease with other organ involvement
American trypanosomiasis
Infection by *Trypanosoma cruzi*
Any condition classifiable to 086.2
086.2 Chagas' disease without mention of
 organ involvement
American trypanosomiasis
Infection by *Trypanosoma cruzi*
086.3 Gambian trypanosomiasis

Gambian sleeping sickness
Infection by *Trypanosoma gambiense*
086.4 Rhodesian trypanosomiasis
Infection by *Trypanosoma rhodesiense*
Rhodesian sleeping sickness
086.5 African trypanosomiasis, unspecified
Sleeping sickness NOS
086.9 Trypanosomiasis, unspecified

087 Relapsing fever
Includes recurrent fever
087.0 Louse-borne
087.1 Tick-borne
087.9 Relapsing fever, unspecified

088 Other arthropod-borne diseases
088.0 Bartonellosis
Carrión's disease
Oroya fever
Verruga peruana
088.8 Other specified arthropod-borne diseases
088.81 Lyme disease
Erythema chronicum migrans
088.89 Other
088.9 Arthropod-borne disease, unspecified

**SYPHILIS AND OTHER SEXUALLY TRANS-
MITTED DISEASES (090 to 099)**
Excludes:
 nonvenereal endemic syphilis (104.0)
 urogenital trichomoniasis (131.0)

090 Congenital syphilis
090.0 Early congenital syphilis, symptomatic
Congenital syphilitic:
 choroiditis
 coryza (chronic)
 hepatomegaly
 mucous patches
 periostitis
 splenomegaly
Syphilitic (congenital):
 epiphysitis
 osteochondritis
 pemphigus
Any congenital syphilitic condition specified as early or manifested less than
 2 years after birth

090.1 Early congenital syphilis, latent
Congenital syphilis without clinical manifestations, with positive serologic reaction and negative spinal fluid test, less than 2 years after birth
090.2 Early congenital syphilis, unspecified
Congenital syphilis NOS, less than 2 years after birth
090.3 Syphilitic interstitial keratitis
Syphilitic keratitis:
  parenchymatous
  punctata profunda
Excludes interstitial keratitis NOS (370.50)
090.4 Juvenile neurosyphilis
Use additional code, if desired, to identify any associated mental disorder
  090.40 Juvenile neurosyphilis, unspecified
  Congenital neurosyphilis
  Dementia paralytica juvenilis
  Juvenile:
    general paresis
    tabes
    taboparesis
  090.41 Congenital syphilitic encephalitis
  090.42 Congenital syphilitic meningitis
  090.49 Other
090.5 Other late congenital syphilis, symptomatic
Gumma due to congenital syphilis
Hutchinson's teeth
Syphilitic saddle nose
Any congenital syphilitic condition specified as late or manifest 2 years or more after birth
090.6 Late congenital syphilis, latent
Congenital syphilis without clinical manifestations, with positive serologic reaction and negative spinal fluid test, 2 years or more after birth
090.7 Late congenital syphilis, unspecified
Congenital syphilis NOS, 2 years or more after birth
090.9 Congenital syphilis, unspecified

091 Early syphilis, symptomatic
Excludes:
  early cardiovascular syphilis (093.0 to 093.9)
  early neurosyphilis (094.0 to 094.9)
091.0 Genital syphilis (primary)

Genital chancre
091.1 Primary anal syphilis
091.2 Other primary syphilis
Primary syphilis of:
  breast
  fingers
  lip
  tonsils
091.3 Secondary syphilis of skin or mucous membranes
Condyloma latum
Secondary syphilis of:
  anus
  mouth
  pharynx
  skin
  tonsils
  vulva
091.4 Adenopathy due to secondary syphilis
Syphilitic adenopathy (secondary)
Syphilitic lymphadenitis (secondary)
091.5 Uveitis due to secondary syphilis
  091.50 Syphilitic uveitis, unspecified
  091.51 Syphilitic chorioretinitis (secondary)
  091.52 Syphilitic iridocyclitis (secondary)
091.6 Secondary syphilis of viscera and bone
  091.61 Secondary syphilitic periostitis
  091.62 Secondary syphilitic hepatitis
  Secondary syphilis of liver
  091.69 Other viscera
091.7 Secondary syphilis, relapse
Secondary syphilis, relapse (treated, untreated)
091.8 Other forms of secondary syphilis
  091.81 Acute syphilitic meningitis (secondary)
  091.82 Syphilitic alopecia
  091.89 Other
091.9 Unspecified secondary syphilis

092 Early syphilis, latent
Includes syphilis (acquired) without clinical manifestations, with positive serologic reaction and negative spinal fluid test, less than 2 years after infection
092.0 Early syphilis, latent, serologic relapse after treatment
092.9 Early syphilis, latent, unspecified

093 Cardiovascular syphilis
  093.0 Aneurysm of aorta, specified as syphilitic
  Dilatation of aorta, specified as syphilitic
  093.1 Syphilitic aortitis
  093.2 Syphilitic endocarditis
    093.20 Valve, unspecified
    Syphilitic ostial coronary disease
    093.21 Mitral valve
    093.22 Aortic valve
    Syphilitic aortic incompetence or stenosis
    093.23 Tricuspid valve
    093.24 Pulmonic valve
  093.8 Other specified cardiovascular syphilis
    093.81 Syphilitic pericarditis
    093.82 Syphilitic myocarditis
    093.89 Other
  093.9 Cardiovascular syphilis, unspecified

094 Neurosyphilis
Use additional code, if desired, to identify any associated mental disorder
  094.0 Tabes dorsalis
  Locomotor ataxia (progressive)
  Posterior spinal sclerosis (syphilitic)
  Tabetic neurosyphilis
  Use additional code, if desired, to identify manifestation as:
    neurogenic arthropathy (Charcot's joint disease, 713.5)
  094.1 General paresis
  Dementia paralytica
  General paralysis (of the insane, progressive)
  Paretic neurosyphilis
  Taboparesis
  094.2 Syphilitic meningitis
  Meningovascular syphilis
  Excludes acute syphilitic meningitis (secondary, 091.81)
  094.3 Asymptomatic neurosyphilis
  094.8 Other specified neurosyphilis
    094.81 Syphilitic encephalitis
    094.82 Syphilitic parkinsonism
    094.83 Syphilitic disseminated retinochoroiditis
    094.84 Syphilitic optic atrophy
    094.85 Syphilitic retrobulbar neuritis
    094.86 Syphilitic acoustic neuritis
    094.87 Syphilitic ruptured cerebral aneurysm

    094.89 Other
  094.9 Neurosyphilis, unspecified (all of 094.9 are of CNS NOS)
  Gumma (syphilitic)
  Syphilis (early, late)
  Syphiloma

095 Other forms of late syphilis, with symptoms
Includes:
  gumma (syphilitic)
  syphilis, late, tertiary, or unspecified stage
  095.0 Syphilitic episcleritis
  095.1 Syphilis of lung
  095.2 Syphilitic peritonitis
  095.3 Syphilis of liver
  095.4 Syphilis of kidney
  095.5 Syphilis of bone
  095.6 Syphilis of muscle
  Syphilitic myositis
  095.7 Syphilis of synovium, tendon, and bursa
  Syphilitic:
    bursitis
    synovitis
  095.8 Other specified forms of late symptomatic syphilis
  Excludes:
    cardiovascular syphilis (093.0 to 093.9)
    neurosyphilis (094.0 to 094.9)
  095.9 Late symptomatic syphilis, unspecified

096 Late syphilis, latent
Syphilis (acquired) without clinical manifestations, with positive serologic reaction and negative spinal fluid test, 2 years or more after infection

097 Other and unspecified syphilis
  097.0 Late syphilis, unspecified
  097.1 Latent syphilis, unspecified
  Positive serologic reaction for syphilis
  097.9 Syphilis, unspecified
  Syphilis (acquired) NOS
  Excludes syphilis NOS causing death under age 2 (090.0)

098 Gonococcal infections
  098.0 Acute, of lower GU tract
  Gonococcal:
    Bartholinitis (acute)

urethritis (acute)
vulvovaginitis (acute)
Gonorrhea (acute):
NOS
GU (tract) NOS
098.1 Acute, of upper GU tract
098.10 Gonococcal infection (acute) of
upper GU tract, site unspecified
098.11 Gonococcal cystitis (acute)
Gonorrhea (acute) of bladder
098.12 Gonococcal prostatitis (acute)
098.13 Gonococcal epididymo-orchitis
(acute)
Gonococcal orchitis (acute)
098.14 Gonococcal seminal vesiculitis
(acute)
Gonorrhea (acute) of seminal vesicle
098.15 Gonococcal cervicitis (acute)
Gonorrhea (acute) of cervix
098.16 Gonococcal endometritis (acute)
Gonorrhea (acute) of uterus
098.17 Gonococcal salpingitis, specified
as acute
098.19 Other
098.2 Chronic, of lower GU tract
Gonococcal:
Bartholinitis
urethritis
vulvovaginitis
Gonorrhea:
NOS
GU (tract)
Any condition classifiable to 098.0
(All of 098.2 are specified as chronic or
with a duration of 2 months or
more.)
098.3 Chronic, of upper GU tract
Includes any condition classifiable to
098.1 stated as chronic or with a duration of 2 months or more
098.30 Chronic gonococcal infection of
upper GU tract, site unspecified
098.31 Gonococcal cystitis, chronic
Any condition classifiable to 098.11,
specified as chronic
Gonorrhea of bladder, chronic
098.32 Gonococcal prostatitis, chronic
Any condition classifiable to 098.12,
specified as chronic
098.33 Gonococcal epididymo-orchitis,
chronic
Any condition classifiable to 098.13,
specified as chronic
Chronic gonococcal orchitis

098.34 Gonococcal seminal vesiculitis,
chronic
Any condition classifiable to 098.14,
specified as chronic
Gonorrhea of seminal vesicle, chronic
098.35 Gonococcal cervicitis, chronic
Any condition classified to 098.15,
specified as chronic
Gonorrhea of cervix, chronic
098.36 Gonococcal endometritis,
chronic
Any condition classifiable to 098.16,
specified as chronic
098.37 Gonococcal salpingitis (chronic)
098.39 Other
098.4 Gonococcal infection of eye
098.40 Gonococcal conjunctivitis (neonatorum)
Gonococcal ophthalmia (neonatorum)
098.41 Gonococcal iridocyclitis
098.42 Gonococcal endophthalmia
098.43 Gonococcal keratitis
098.49 Other
098.5 Gonococcal infection of joint
098.50 Gonococcal arthritis
Gonococcal infection of joint NOS
098.51 Gonococcal synovitis and tenosynovitis
098.52 Gonococcal bursitis
098.53 Gonococcal spondylitis
098.59 Other
Gonococcal rheumatism
098.6 Gonococcal infection of pharynx
098.7 Gonococcal infection of anus and
rectum
Gonococcal proctitis
098.8 Gonococcal infection of other specified sites
098.81 Gonococcal keratosis (kerato-
derma blennorrhagicum)
098.82 Gonococcal meningitis
098.83 Gonococcal pericarditis
098.84 Gonococcal endocarditis
098.85 Other gonococcal heart disease
098.86 Gonococcal peritonitis
098.89 Other
Gonococcemia

099 Other venereal diseases
099.0 Chancroid
Bubo (inguinal):
chancroidal
due to *Haemophilus ducreyi*

Chancre:
  Ducrey's
  simple
  soft
Ulcus molle (cutis, skin)
099.1 Lymphogranuloma venereum
  Climatic or tropical bubo
  Durand-Nicolas-Favre disease
  Esthiomene
  Lymphogranuloma inguinale
099.2 Granuloma inguinale
  Donovanosis
  Granuloma pudendi (ulcerating)
  Granuloma venereum
  Pudendal ulcer
099.3 Reiter's disease
  Reiter's syndrome
099.4 Other nongonococcal urethritis
  Nonspecific and nongonococcal urethri-
    tis, so stated
099.8 Other specified venereal diseases
099.9 Venereal disease, unspecified

OTHER SPIROCHETAL DISEASES (100 to 104)

100 Leptospirosis
  100.0 Leptospirosis icterohemorrhagica
    Leptospiral or spirochetal jaundice (hem-
      orrhagic)
    Weil's disease
  100.8 Other specified leptospiral infections
    100.81 Leptospiral meningitis (aseptic)
    100.89 Other
      Fever:
        Fort Bragg
        pretibial
        swamp
      Infection by *Leptospira:*
        australis
        bataviae
        pyrogenes
  100.9 Leptospirosis, unspecified

101 Vincent's angina
  Acute necrotizing ulcerative:
    gingivitis
    stomatitis
  Fusospirochetal pharyngitis
  Spirochetal stomatitis
  Trench mouth

Vincent's:
  gingivitis
  infection (any site)

102 Yaws
Includes:
  frambesia
  pian
  102.0 Initial lesions
    Chancre of yaws
    Frambesia, initial or primary
    Initial frambesial ulcer
    Mother yaw
  102.1 Multiple papillomata and wet crab
    yaws
    Butter yaws
    Frambesioma
    Pianoma
    Plantar of palmar papilloma of yaws
  102.2 Other early skin lesions
    Early yaws (cutaneous, macular, papular,
      maculopapular, micropapular)
    Frambeside of early yaws
    Cutaneous yaws, less than 5 years after
      infection
  102.3 Hyperkeratosis
    Ghoul hand
    Hyperkeratosis, palmar or plantar (early,
      late) due to yaws
    Worm-eaten soles
  102.4 Gummata and ulcers
    Nodular late yaws (ulcerated)
    Gummatous frambeside
  102.5 Gangosa
    Rhinopharyngitis mutilans
  102.6 Bone and joint lesions
    Goundou of yaws (late)
    Gumma, bone of yaws (late)
    Gummatous osteitis or periostitis of
      yaws (late)
    Hydrarthrosis of yaws (early, late)
    Osteitis of yaws (early, late)
    Periostitis (hypertrophic) of yaws (early,
      late)
  102.7 Other manifestations
    Juxta-articular nodules of yaws
    Mucosal yaws
  102.8 Latent yaws
    Yaws without clinical manifestations,
      with positive serology
  102.9 Yaws, unspecified

103 Pinta
103.0 Primary lesions of pinta (carate)
Chancre (primary)
Papule (primary)
Pintid
103.1 Intermediate lesions of pinta (carate)
Erythematous plaques
Hyperchromic lesions
Hyperkeratosis
103.2 Late lesions of pinta (carate)
Cardiovascular lesions
Skin lesions:
achromic
cicatricial
dyschromic
Vitiligo
103.3 Mixed lesions
Achromic and hyperchromic skin lesions
of pinta (carate)
103.9 Pinta, unspecified

104 Other spirochetal infection
104.0 Nonvenereal endemic syphilis
Bejel
Njovera
104.8 Other specified spirochetal infections
Excludes:
relapsing fever (087.0 to 087.9)
syphilis (090.7 to 097.9)
104.9 Spirochetal infection, unspecified

MYCOSES (110 to 118)
Use additional code, if desired, to identify
manifestation as:
arthropathy (711.6)
meningitis (321.0 to 321.1)
otitis externa (380.15)
Excludes infection by Actinomycetales, such
as species of *Actinomyces, Actinomadura, Nocardia, Streptomyces* (039.0 to
039.9)

110 Dermatophytosis
Includes:
infection by species of:
Epidermophyton
Microsporum
Trichophyton
tinea, any type except those in 111
110.0 Of scalp and beard
Kerion
Sycosis, mycotic

Trichophytic tinea (black dot tinea), scalp
110.1 Of nail
Dermatophytic onychia
Onychomycosis
Tinea unguium
110.2 Of hand
Tinea manuum
110.3 Of groin and perianal area
Dhobie itch
Eczema marginatum
Tinea cruris
110.4 Of foot
Athlete's foot
Tinea pedis
110.5 Of the body
Herpes circinatus
Tinea imbricata (tokelau)
110.6 Deep seated dermatophytosis
Granuloma trichophyticum
Majocchi's granuloma
110.8 Of other specified sites
110.9 Of unspecified site
Favus NOS
Microsporic tinea NOS
Ringworm NOS

111 Dermatomycosis, other and unspecified
111.0 Pityriasis versicolor
Infection by *Malassezia* (Pityrosporum)
furfur
Tinea flava
Tinea versicolor
111.1 Tinea nigra
Infection by *Cladosporium* species
Keratomycosis nigricans
Microsporosis nigra
Pityriasis nigra
Tinea palmaris nigra
111.2 Tinea blanca
Infection by *Trichosporon (beigelii) cuta-
neum*
White piedra
111.3 Black piedra
Infection by *Piedraia hortaie*
111.8 Other specified dermatomycoses
111.9 Dermatomycosis, unspecified

112 Candidiasis
Includes infection by *Candida* species
moniliasis
Excludes neonatal monilial infection (771.7)
112.0 Of mouth
Thrush (oral)

112.1 Of vulva and vagina
Candidal vulvovaginitis
Monilial vulvovaginitis
112.2 Of other urogenital sites
Candidal balanitis
112.3 Of skin and nails
Candidal intertrigo
Candidal onychia
Candidal perionyxis (paronychia)
112.4 Of lung
Candidal pneumonia
112.5 Disseminated
Systemic candidiasis
112.8 Of other specified sites
  112.81 Candidal endocarditis
  112.82 Candidal otitis externa
Otomycosis in moniliasis
  112.83 Candidal meningitis
  112.89 Other
112.9 Of unspecified site

114 Coccidioidomycosis
Includes:
infection by *Coccidioides (immitis)*
Posada-Wernicke disease
114.0 Primary coccidioidomycosis (pulmonary)
Coccidioidomycotic pneumonitis
Desert rheumatism
Pulmonary coccidioidomycosis
San Joaquin Valley fever
114.1 Primary extrapulmonary coccidioidomycosis
Chancriform syndrome
Primary cutaneous coccidioidomycosis
114.2 Coccidioidal meningitis
114.3 Other forms of progressive coccidioidomycosis
Coccidioidal granuloma
Disseminated coccidioidomycosis
114.9 Coccidioidomycosis, unspecified

115 Histoplasmosis
The following fifth-digit subclassification is for use with category 115:
0 = without mention of manifestation
1 = meningitis
2 = retinitis
3 = pericarditis
4 = endocarditis
5 = pneumonia
9 = other

115.0 Infection by *Histoplasma capsulatum*
American histoplasmosis
Darling's disease
Reticuloendothelial cytomycosis
Small form histoplasmosis
115.1 Infection by *Histoplasma duboisii*
African histoplasmosis
Large form histoplasmosis
115.9 Histoplasmosis, unspecified
Histoplasmosis NOS

116 Blastomycotic infection
116.0 Blastomycosis
Blastomycotic dermatitis
Chicago disease
Cutaneous blastomycosis
Disseminated blastomycosis
Gilchrist's disease
Infection by *Blastomyces (Ajellomyces) dermatitidis*
North American blastomycosis
Primary pulmonary blastomycosis
116.1 Paracoccidiodomycosis
Brazilian blastomycosis
Infection by *Paracoccidioides (Blastomyces) brasiliensis*
Lutz-Splendore-Almeida disease
Mucocutaneous-lymphangitic paracoccidioidomycosis
Pulmonary paracoccidioidomycosis
South American blastomycosis
Visceral paracoccidioidomycosis
116.2 Lobomycosis
Infections by *Loboa (Blastomyces) loboi*
Keloidal blastomycosis
Lobo's disease

117 Other mycoses
117.0 Rhinosporidiosis
Infection by *Rhinosporidium seeberi*
117.1 Sporotrichosis
Cutaneous sporotrichosis
Disseminated sporotrichosis
Infection by *Sporothrix (Sporotrichum) schenckii*
Lymphocutaneous sporotrichosis
Pulmonary sporotrichosis
Sporotrichosis of the bones
117.2 Chromoblastomycosis
Chromomycosis

Infection by *Cladosporidium carrionii,
Fonsecaea compactum, F. pedrosoi,
Phialophora verrucosa*
117.3 Aspergillosis
Infection by *Aspergillus* species, mainly
A. fumigatus, A. flavus group, *A. ter-
reus* group
117.4 Mycotic mycetomas
Infection by various genera and species
of Ascomycetes and Deuteromy-
cetes, such as *Acremonium (Cepha-
losporium) falciforme, Neotestundina
rosatii, Madurella grisea, Madurella
mycetomii, Pyrenochaeta romeroi,
Zopfia (Leptosphaeria) senegalensis*
Madura foot, mycotic
Maduromycosis, mycotic
Excludes actinomycotic mycetomas
(039.0 to 039.9)
117.5 Cryptococcosis
Busse-Buschke's disease
European cryptococcosis
Infection by *Cryptococcus neoformans*
Pulmonary cryptococcosis
Systemic cryptococcosis
Torula
117.6 Allescheriosis (Petriellidosis)
Infection by *Allescheria (Petriellidium)
boydii (Monosporium apiospermum)*
Excludes mycotic mycetoma (117.4)
117.7 Zygomycosis (Phycomycosis or Mu-
cormycosis)
Infection by species of *Absidia, Basi-
diobolus, Conidiobolus, Cunningha-
mella, Entomophthora, Mucor,
Rhizopus, Saksenaea*
117.8 Infection by dematiacious fungi
(Phaehyphomycosis)
Infection by dermatiacious fungi, such
as *Cladosporium trichoides (ban-
tianum), Dreschlera hawaiiensis, Phialophora gougerotii, Phialophora
jeanselmi*
117.9 Other and unspecified mycoses

118 Opportunistic mycoses
Infection of skin, subcutaneous tissue, or organs by a wide variety of fungi generally
considered to be pathogenic to compromised hosts only (such as infection by
species of *Alternaria, Dreschlera, Fusar-
ium)*

HELMINTHIASES (120 to 129)

120 Schistosomiasis (bilharziasis)
120.0 *Schistosoma haematobium*
Vesical schistosomiasis NOS
120.1 *Schistosoma mansoni*
Intestinal schistosomiasis NOS
120.2 *Schistosoma japonicum*
Asiatic schistosomiasis NOS
Katayama disease or fever
120.3 Cutaneous
Cercarial dermatitis
Infection by cercariae of *Schistosoma*
Schistosome dermatitis
Swimmers' itch
120.8 Other specified schistosomiasis
Infection by *Schistosoma:*
bovis
intercalatum
mattheii
Infection by *Schistosoma spindale*
Schistosomiasis chestermani
120.9 Schistosomiasis unspecified
Blood flukes NOS
Hemic distomiasis

121 Other trematode infections
121.0 Opisthorchiasis
Infection by:
cat liver fluke
*Opisthorchis (felineus, tenuicollis,
viverrini)*
121.1 Clonorchiasis
Biliary cirrhosis due to clonorchiasis
Chinese liver fluke disease
Hepatic distomiasis due to *Clonorchis si-
nensis*
Oriental liver fluke disease
121.2 Paragonimiasis
Infection by Paragonimus
Lung fluke disease (oriental)
Pulmonary distomiasis
121.3 Fascioliasis
Infection by *Fasciola:*
gigantica
hepatica
Liver flukes NOS
Sheep liver fluke infection
121.4 Fasciolopsiasis
Infection by *Fasciolopsis (buski)*
Intestinal distomiasis

121.5 Metagonimiasis
Infection by *Metagonimus yokogawai*
121.6 Heterophyiasis
Infection by:
  Heterophyes heterophyes
  Stellantchasmus falcatus
121.8 Other specified trematode infections
Infection by:
  Dicrocoelium dendriticum
  Echinostoma ilocanum
  Gastrodiscoides hominis
121.9 Trematode infection, unspecified
Distomiasis NOS
Fluke disease NOS

122 Echinococcosis
Includes:
  echinococciasis
  hydatid disease
  hydatidosis
122.0 *Echinococcus granulosus* infection
  of liver
122.1 *Echinococcus granulosus* infection
  of lung
122.2 *Echinococcus granulosus* infection
  of thyroid
122.3 *Echinococcus granulosus* infection,
  other
122.4 *Echinococcus granulosus* infection,
  unspecified
122.5 *Echinococcus multilocularis* infection of liver
122.6 *Echinococcus multilocularis* infection, other
122.7 *Echinococcus multilocularis* infection, unspecified
122.8 Echinococcosis, unspecified, of liver
122.9 Echinococcosis, other and unspecified

123 Other cestode infection
123.0 *Taenia solium* infection, intestinal
  form
Pork tapeworm (adult, infection)
123.1 Cysticercosis
Cysticerciasis
Infection by *Cysticercus cellulosae* (larval form of *Taenia solium)*
123.2 *Taenia saginata* infection
Beef tapeworm (infection)
Infection by *Taeniarhynchus saginatus*
123.3 Taeniasis, unspecified
123.4 Diphyllobothriasis, intestinal

Diphyllobothrium (adult, *latum, pacifi-
  cum)* infection
Fish tapeworm (infection)
123.5 Sparganosis (larval diphylloboth-
  riasis)
Infection by:
  Diphyllobothrium larvae
  Sparganum (mansoni, proliferum)
  Spirometra larvae
123.6 Hymenolepiasis
Dwarf tapeworm (infection)
Hymenolepis (diminuta, nana) infection
Rat tapeworm (infection)
123.8 Other specified cestode infection
  Diplogonoporus (grandis)
  Dipylidium (caninum)
  Dog tapeworm (infection)
123.9 Cestode infection, unspecified
Tapeworm (infection) NOS

124 Trichinosis
Trichinella spiralis infection
Trichinellosis
Trichiniasis

125 Filarial infection and dracontiasis
125.0 Bancroftian filariasis
due to *Wuchereria bancrofti:*
  Chyluria
  Elephantiasis
  Infection
  Lymphadenitis
  Lymphangitis
  Wuchereriasis
125.1 Malayan filariasis
due to *Brugia (Wuchereria) malayi:*
  Brugia filariasis
  Chyluria
  Elephantiasis
  Infection
  Lymphadenitis
  Lymphangitis
125.2 Loiasis
Eyeworm disease of Africa
Loa loa infection
125.3 Onchocerciasis
Onchocerca volvulus infection
Onchocercosis
125.4 Dipetalonemiasis
Infection by:
  Acanthocheilonema perstans
  Dipetalonema perstans

125.5 *Mansonella ozzardi* infection
 Filariasis ozzardi
125.6 Other specified filariasis
 Dirofilaria infection
 Infection by:
   Acanthocheilonema streptocerca
   Dipetalonema streptocerca
125.7 Dracontiasis
 Guinea-worm infection
 Infection by *Dracunculus medinensis*
125.9 Unspecified filariasis

126 Ancylostomiasis and necatoriasis
Includes:
 cutaneous *larva migrans* due to *Ancylostoma* hookworm (disease, infection)
 uncinariasis
126.0 *Ancylostoma duodenale*
126.1 *Necator americanus*
126.2 *Ancylostoma braziliense*
126.3 *Ancylostoma ceylanicum*
126.8 Other specified *Ancylostoma*
126.9 Ancylostomiasis and necatoriasis,
  unspecified
 Creeping eruption NOS
 Cutaneous *larva migrans* NOS

127 Other intestinal helminthiases
127.0 Ascariasis
 Ascaridiasis
 Infection by *Ascaris lumbricoides*
 Roundworm infection
127.1 *Anisakiasis*
 Infection by *Anisakis* larva
127.2 Strongyloidiasis
 Infection by *Strongyloides stercoralis*
 Excludes trichostrongyliasis (127.6)
127.3 Trichuriasis
 Infection by *Trichuris trichiuria*
 Trichocephaliasis
 Whipworm (disease, infection)
127.4 Enterobiasis
 Infection by *Enterobius vermicularis*
 Oxyuriasis
 Oxyuris vermicularis infection
 Pinworm (disease, infection)
 Threadworm infection
127.5 Capillariasis
 Infection by *Capillaria philippinensis*
 Excludes infection by *Capillaria hepatica*
  (128.8)
127.6 Trichostrongyliasis
 Infection by *Trichostrongylus* species

127.7 Other specified intestinal helminthiasis
 Infection by:
   Oesophagostomum apiostomum and
    related species
   Ternidens diminutus
   other specified intestinal helminth
 Physalopteriasis
127.8 Mixed intestinal helminthiasis
 Infection by intestinal helminths classified to more than one of the categories 120.0 to 127.7
 Mixed helminthiasis NOS
127.9 Intestinal helminthiasis, unspecified

128 Other and unspecified helminthiases
128.0 Toxocariasis
 Larva migrans visceralis
 Toxocara (canis, cati) infection
 Visceral *larva migrans* syndrome
128.1 Gnathostomiasis
 Infection by *Gnathostoma spinigerum*
  and related species
128.8 Other specified helminthiasis
 Infection by:
   Angiostrongylus cantonensis
   Capillaria hepatica
   other specified helminth
128.9 Helminth infection, unspecified
 Helminthiasis NOS
 Worms NOS

129 Intestinal parasitism, unspecified

**OTHER INFECTIOUS AND PARASITIC DIS-
EASES (130 to 136)**

130 Toxoplasmosis
Includes:
 infection by *Toxoplasma gondii* toxoplasmosis (acquired)
Excludes congenital toxoplasmosis (771.2)
130.0 Meningoencephalitis due to toxoplasmosis
 Encephalitis due to acquired toxoplasmosis
130.1 Conjunctivitis due to toxoplasmosis
130.2 Chorioretinitis due to toxoplasmosis
 Focal retinochoroiditis due to acquired
  toxoplasmosis
130.3 Myocarditis due to toxoplasmosis
130.4 Pneumonitis due to toxoplasmosis

130.5 Hepatitis due to toxoplasmosis
130.7 Toxoplasmosis of other specified
sites
130.8 Multisystemic disseminated toxoplasmosis
Toxoplasmosis of multiple sites
130.9 Toxoplasmosis, unspecified

131 Trichomoniasis
Includes infection due to *Trichomonas (vaginalis)*
131.0 Urogenital trichomoniasis
131.00 Urogenital trichomoniasis, unspecified (trichomonal or due to *Trichomonas [vaginalis]*)
Fluor (vaginalis)
Leukorrhea (vaginalis)
131.01 Trichomonal vulvovaginitis
Vaginitis, trichomonal or due to *Trichomonas (vaginalis)*
131.02 Trichomonal urethritis
131.03 Trichomonal prostatitis
131.09 Other
131.8 Other specified sites
131.9 Trichomoniasis, unspecified

132 Pediculosis and phthirus infestation
132.0 *Pediculus capitis* (head louse)
132.1 *Pediculus corporis* (body louse)
132.2 *Phthirus pubis* (pubic louse)
Pediculus pubis
132.3 Mixed infestation
132.9 Pediculosis, unspecified

133 Acariasis
133.0 Scabies
Infestation by *Sarcoptes scabiei*
Norwegian scabies
Sarcoptic itch
133.8 Other acariasis
Chiggers
Infestation by:
Demodex folliculorum
Trombicula
133.9 Acariasis, unspecified
Infestation by mites NOS

134 Other infestation
134.0 Myiasis
Infestation by:
Dermatobia (hominis)
fly larvae
Gasterophilus (intestinalis)

maggots
Oestrus ovis

135 Sarcoidosis
Besnier-Boeck-Schaumann disease
Lupoid (miliary) of Boeck
Lupus pernio (Besnier)
Lymphogranulomatosis, benign
Sarcoid (any site)
Uveoparotid fever

**136 Other and unspecified infectious and
parasitic diseases**
136.0 Ainhum
Dactylolysis spontanea
136.1 Behçet's syndrome
136.2 Infections by free-living amebae
Meningoencephalitis due to *Naegleria*
136.3 Pneumocystosis
Pneumonia due to *Pneumocystis carinii*
136.4 Psorospermiasis
136.5 Sarcosporidiosis
Infection by *Sarcocystis lindemanni*
136.8 Other specified infectious and parasitic diseases
Candiru infestation

**LATE EFFECTS OF INFECTIOUS AND PARA-
SITIC DISEASES (137 to 139)**

137 Late effects of tuberculosis
137.0 Late effects of respiratory or unspecified tuberculosis
137.1 Late effects of CNS tuberculosis
137.2 Late effects of GU tuberculosis
137.3 Late effects of tuberculosis on
bones and joints
137.4 Effects of tuberculosis of other specified organs

138 Late effects of acute poliomyelitis
Note: This category is to be used to indicate
conditions classifiable to 045 as the
cause of late effects, which are themselves classified elsewhere.

**139 Late effects of other infectious and par-
asitic diseases**
139.0 Late effects of viral encephalitis
139.1 Late effects of trachoma
139.8 Late effects of other and unspecified
infectious and parasitic diseases

Index

i refers to an illustration; t refers to a table

i refers to an illustration; t refers to a table

i refers to an illustration; t refers to a table